FOURTEEN LESSONS

in

Yogi Philosophy

and

Oriental Occultism

By YOGI RAMACHARAKA

Author of "Science of Breath," "Hatha Yoga," etc.

⌒

"Know, O disciple! that those who have passed
through the silence, and felt its peace, and retained
its strength, they long that you shall pass through
it also. Therefore, in the Hall of Learning, when
he is capable of entering there, the disciple will
always find his master." — *Light on the Path.*

⌒

The Yoga Publication Society
Chicago 10, Illinois

ISBN #0-911662-01-4

TABLE OF CONTENTS.

TABLE OF CONTENTS—Continued.

THE FIRST LESSON.

THE FIRST THREE PRINCIPLES.

IT is with no ordinary feelings that we address ourselves to our students of the Yogi class of 1904. We see, as they perhaps do not, that to many of them this series of lessons will be as seed planted in fertile soil, which will in due time put forth sprouts which will force their way gradually into the sunlight of consciousness, where they will put forth leaves, blossom, and fruit. Many of the fragments of truth which will be presented to you will not be recognized by you at this time, but in years to come you will recognize the verity of the impressions which will be conveyed to you in these lessons, and then, and then only, will you make these truths your own.

We intend to speak to you just as if you were gathered before us in person, and as if we were standing before you in the flesh. We feel sure that the bond of sympathy between us will soon grow so strong and real that as you read our words you will feel our presence almost as strongly as if we were with you in person. We will be with you in spirit, and, according to our philosophy, the student who is in harmonious sympathy with his teachers really establishes a psychic connection with them, and is in consequence enabled to grasp the "spirit" of the teaching and to receive the benefit of the teacher's thought in a degree impossible to one who merely reads the words in cold print.

We are sure that the members of the class of 1904 will get into harmony with each other, and with us, from the very start, and that we will obtain results that will surprise even ourselves, and that the term of the class will mark a wonderful spiritual growth and unfoldment for many of the class. This result would be impossible were the class composed of the general public, in which the adverse thought vibrations of many would counteract, or at least retard, the impelling force generated in the minds of those who are in sympathy with the work. But we will not have this obstacle to overcome, as the class has been recruited only from that class of students who are interested in the occult. The announcements sent out by us have been worded in such a way as to attract the attention only of those for whom they were intended. The mere sensation-hunters and the "faddists" have not been attracted by our call, while those for whom the call was intended have heard and have hastened to communicate with us. As the poet has sung: "Where I pass, all my children know me." The members of the class having been attracted to us, and we to them, will form a harmonious body working with us to the common end of self-improvement, growth, development, and unfoldment. The spirit of harmony and unity of purpose will do much for us, and the united thought of the class, coupled with our own, will be a tower of strength, and each student will receive the benefit of it, and will be strengthened and sustained thereby.

We will follow the system of instruction of the East, rather than that of the Western world. In the East, the teacher does not stop to "prove" each statement or theory as he makes or advances it; nor does he make a blackboard demonstration of spiritual truths; nor does he argue with his class or invite discussion. On the contrary, his teaching is authoritative, and he proceeds to deliver his message to his students as it was delivered to him, without stopping to see whether they all agree with him. He does not care whether his statements are accepted as truth by all, for he feels sure that those who are ready for the truth which he teaches will intuitively recognize it, and as for the others, if they are not prepared to receive the truth, no amount of argument will help matters. When a soul is ready for a spiritual truth, and that truth, or a part of it, is uttered in its presence or presented to its attention by means of writings, it will intuitively recognize and appropriate it. The Eastern teacher knows that much of his teaching is but the planting of seed, and that for every idea which the student grasps at first there will be a hundred which will come into the field of conscious recognition only after the lapse of time.

We do not mean that the Eastern teachers insist upon the student blindly accepting every truth that is presented to him. On the contrary, they instruct the pupil to accept as truth only that which he can prove for himself, as no truth is truth to one until he can prove it by his own experiments. But the student is taught that before many truths may be so proven he must develop and unfold. The teacher asks only that the student have confidence in him as a pointer-out of the way, and he says, in effect, to the student: "This is the way; enter upon it, and on the path you will find the things of which I have taught you; handle them, weigh them, measure them, taste them, and know for yourself. When you reach any point of the path you will know as much of it as did I or any other soul at that particular stage of the journey; but until you reach a particular point, you must either accept the statements of those who have gone before or reject the whole subject of that particular point. Accept nothing as final until you have proven it; but, if you are wise, you will profit by the advice and experience of those who have gone before. Every man must learn by experience, but men may serve others as pointers of the way. At each stage of the journey it will be found that those who have progressed a little further on the way have left signs and marks and guide-posts for those who follow. The wise man will take advantage of these signs. I do not ask for blind faith, but only for confidence until you are able to demonstrate for yourselves the truths I am passing on to you, as they were passed on to me, by those who went before.

We ask the student to have patience. Many things which will appear dark to him at first will be made clear as we progress.

THE CONSTITUTION OF MAN.

Man is a far more complete being than is generally imagined. He has not only a body and a soul, but he is a spirit possessing a soul, which soul has several vehicles for expression, these several vehicles being of different degrees of density, the body being the lowest form of expression. These different vehicles manifest upon different "planes," such as the "physical plane," the "astral plane," etc., all of which will be explained as we proceed.

The real self is pure spirit—a spark of the divine fire. This spirit is encased within numerous sheaths, which prevent its full expression. As man advances in development, his consciousness passes from the lower planes to the higher, and he becomes more and more aware of his higher nature.

The spirit contains within it all potentialities, and as man progresses he unfolds new powers, new qualities, into the light.

The Yogi philosophy teaches that man is composed of seven principles—is a sevenfold creature. The best way to think of man is to realize that the spirit is the real self, and that the lower principles are but confining sheaths. Man may manifest upon seven planes, that is, the highly developed man, as the majority of men of this age can manifest only upon the lower planes, the higher planes not having as yet been reached by them, although every man, no matter how undeveloped, possesses the seven principles potentially. The first five planes have been attained by many, the sixth by a few, the seventh by practically none of this race at this time.

The Seven Principles of Man.

The seven principles of man, as known to the Yogi philosophy, are herewith stated, English terms being substituted for Sanscrit words, so far as may be:

7. *Spirit.*
6. *Spiritual-Mind.*
5. *Intellect.*
4. *Instinctive-Mind.*
3. *Prana, or Vital Force.*
2. *Astral Body.*
1. *Physical Body.*

We will briefly run over the general nature of each of these seven principles, that the student may understand future references to them; but we will defer our detailed treatment of the subject until later on in the lessons.

1. *The Physical Body.*

Of all the seven principles of man, the physical body is of course the most apparent. It is the lowest in the scale, and is the crudest manifestation of the man. But this does not mean that the physical should be despised or neglected. On the contrary, it is a most necessary principle for the growth of man in his present stage of development—the temple of the living Spirit—and it should be carefully tended and cared for in order to render it a more perfect instrument. We have but to look around us and see how the physical bodies of different men show the different degrees of development under mental control. It is a duty of each developed man to train his body to the highest degree of perfection in order that it may be used to advantage. The body should be kept in good health and condition and trained to obey the orders of the mind, rather than to rule the mind, as is so often the case. The care of the body, under the intelligent control of the mind, is an important branch of Yogi philosophy, and is known as "Hatha Yoga." We are preparing a little text-book upon "Hatha Yoga," which will soon be ready for the press, that will give the Yogi teachings upon this most important branch of self-development. The Yogi philosophy teaches that the physical body is built up of cells, each cell containing within it a miniature "life," which controls its action. These "lives" are really bits of intelligent mind of a certain degree of growth, which enable the cells to perform their work properly. These bits of intelligence are, of course, subordinate to the control of the central mind of the man, and will readily obey orders from headquarters, given either subconsciously or consciously. These cell intelligences manifest a perfect adaptation for their particular work. The selective action of the cells, extracting from the blood the nourishment needed and rejecting that which is not required, is an instance of this intelligence. The process of digestion, assimilation, etc., shows the intelligence of the cells, either separately or collectively in groups. The healing of wounds, the rush of the cells to the points where they are most needed, and hundreds of other examples known to the student of physiology, all mean to the Yogi student examples of the "life" within each atom. Each atom is to the Yogi a living thing, leading its own independent life. These atoms combine into groups for some end, and the group manifests a group-intelligence, as long as it remains a group; these groups again combining in turn, and forming bodies of a more complex nature, which serve as vehicles for higher forms of consciousness.

When death comes to the physical body the cells separate and scatter, and that which we call decay sets in. The force which has held the cells together is withdrawn, and it becomes free to go its own way and form new combinations. Some go into the body of the plants in the vicinity, and eventually find themselves again in the body of an animal; others remain in the organism of the plant; others remain in the ground for a time, but the life of the atom means incessant and constant change. As a leading writer has said: "Death is but an aspect of life, and the destruction of one material form is but a prelude to the building up of another."

We will not devote further space to the consideration of the physical, as that is a subject by itself, and, then, our students are no doubt anxious to be led into subjects with which they are not quite so familiar. So we will leave this first principle and pass on to the second, wishing, however, again to remind the student that the first step in Yogi development consists of the mastery of the physical body and its care and attention. We will have more to say of this subject before we are through with this course.

The Astral Body.

This second principle of man is not nearly so well known as its physical brother, although it is closely connected with the latter and is its exact counterpart in appearance. The astral body has been known to people in all ages, and has given rise to many superstitions and mysteries, owing to a lack of knowledge of its nature. It has been called the "ethereal body"; the "fluidic body"; the "double"; the "wraith"; the "Doppelganger," etc. It is composed of matter of a finer quality than that composing our physical bodies, but matter none the less. In order to give you a clearer idea of what we mean, we will call your attention to water, which manifests in several well-known forms. Water at a certain temperature is known as ice, a hard, solid substance; at a little higher temperature it assumes its best-known form, which we call "water"; at a still higher temperature it escapes in the form of a vapor which we call "steam," although the real steam is invisible to the human eye, and becomes apparent only when it mixes with the air and has its temperature lowered a little, when it becomes vapor visible to the eye, and which vapor we call "steam."

The astral body is the best counterpart of the physical body and may be separated from it under certain circumstances. Ordinarily, conscious separation is a matter of considerable difficulty, but in persons of a certain degree of psychical development the astral body may be detached and often goes on long journeys. To the clairvoyant vision the astral body is seen looking exactly like its counterpart, the phys ical body, and united to it by a slender silken cord.

The astral body exists some time after the death of the person to whom it belongs, and under certain circumstances it is visible to living persons, and is called a "ghost." There are other means whereby the spirits of those who have passed on may become manifest, and the astral shell which is sometimes seen after it has been sloughed off by the soul which has passed on is in such cases nothing more than a corpse of finer matter than its physical counterpart. In such cases it is possessed of no life or intelligence, and is nothing more than a cloud seen in the sky bearing a resemblance to a human form. It is a shell, nothing more. The astral body of a dying person is sometimes projected by an earnest desire, and is at such times seen by friends and relatives with whom he is in sympathy. There are many cases of this kind on record, and the student probably is aware of occurrences of this kind. We will have more to say about the astral body and astral shells in other lessons in this course. We will have occasion to go into further detail when we reach the subject of the astral plane, and, in fact, the astral body will form a part of several lessons.

The astral body is invisible to the ordinary eye, but is readily perceived by those having clairvoyant power of a certain degree. Under certain circumstances the astral body of a living person may be seen by friends and others, the mental condition of the persons and the observer having much to do with the matter. Of course, the trained and developed occultist is able to project his astral body consciously, and may make it appear at will; but such powers are rare and are acquired only after a certain stage of development is reached.

The adept sees the astral body rising from the physical body as the hour of death approaches. It is seen hovering over the physical body, to which it is bound by a slender thread. When the thread snaps the person is dead, and the soul passes on carrying with it the astral body, which in turn is discarded as the physical body has been before. It must be remembered that the astral body is merely a finer grade of matter, and that it is merely a vehicle for the soul, just as is the physical, and that both are discarded at the proper time. The astral body, like the physical, disintegrates after the death of the person, and persons of a psychic nature sometimes see the dissolving fragments around cemeteries, in the shape of violet light.

We are merely calling attention to the different vehicles of the soul of man, his seven principles, and we must hasten on to the next principle. We would like to speak to you of the interesting phenomenon of the ego leaving the physical body in the astral body while one is "asleep." We would like to tell you just what occurs during sleep, and how one may give orders to his astral self to gain

certain information or to work out certain problems while he is wrapped in sleep, but that belongs
to another phase of our subject, and we must pass
on after merely whetting your appetite. We wish
you to get these seven principles well fixed in your
mind, so that you may be able to understand the
terms when we use them later on.

3. *Prana, or Vital Force.*

We have said something of Prana in our little
book, "The Science of Breath," which many of you
have read. As we said in that book, Prana is universal energy, but in our consideration of it we will
confine ourselves to that manifestation of Prana
which we call vital force. This vital force is found
in all forms of life—from the amœba to man—from
the most elementary form of plant life to the highest form of animal life. Prana is all-pervading. It
is found in all things having life, and as the occult
philosophy teaches that life is in all things—in every
atom—the apparent lifelessness of some things being
only a lesser degree of manifestation, we may understand that Prana is everywhere, in everything.
Prana is not the Ego, but is merely a form of energy
used by the Ego in its material manifestation.
When the Ego departs from the physical body, in
what we call "death," the Prana, being no longer
under the control of the Ego, responds only to the
orders of the individual atoms or their groups,

which have formed the physical body, and as the physical body disintegrates and is resolved back to its orginal elements, each atom takes with it sufficient Prana to enable it to form new combinations, the unused Prana returning to the great universal storehouse from whence it came. Prana is in all forms of matter, and yet it is not matter—it is the energy or force which animates matter. We have gone into the matter of Prana in our little book previously referred to, and we do not wish to take up the students' time in repeating what we said there.

But before taking up the next principle, we wish to direct the student's attention to the fact that Prana is the force underlying magnetic healing, much of mental healing, absent treatment, etc. That which has been spoken of by many as human magnetism is really Prana.

In "Science of Breath," we have given you directions for increasing the Prana in your system; distributing it over the body, strengthening each part and organ and stimulating every cell. It may be directed toward relieving pain in one's self and others by sending to the affected part a supply of Prana extracted from the air. It may be projected to a distance so far as to affect other persons. The thought of the projector sends forth and colors the Prana gathered for the purpose, and finds lodgment in the psychic organism of the patient. Like the

Marconi waves it is invisible to the eye of man (with the exception of certain persons who have attained a high degree of clairvoyant power) ; it passes through intervening obstacles and seeks the person attuned to receive it.

This transferring of Prana under the direction of the will is the underlying principle of thought transference, telepathy, etc. One may surround himself with an aura of Prana, colored with strong positive thought, which will enable him to resist the adverse thought waves of others, and which will enable him to live serene in an atmosphere of antagonistic and inharmonious thought.

We advise students to re-read that portion of "Science of Breath" which deals with the use of Prana. We propose going into great detail regarding this phase of the subject, during the course of these lessons, but "Science of Breath" gives a good fundamental idea of the nature of Prana and the methods of its use, and students will do well to refresh their minds on this subject.

We do not wish to weary you by this description of each of the seven principles, and we are aware that you are impatient to enter into the more interesting phases of the subject. But it is absolutely necessary that you obtain a clear idea of these seven principles, in order that you may understand that which follows, and to obviate the necessity of your being "sent back" to relearn the lesson which you have "skipped." We had this idea in mind when we started this class in November, 1903, instead of waiting until January, 1904, and we give you the November and December lessons as "good measure," so as to be able to reach the more interesting part of the subject by the January lesson.

We will leave the subject of Prana and will pass on to the next principle; but we trust that you will not leave this part of the lesson until you have acquired a clear idea of Prana and its qualities and uses. Study your "Science of Breath" until you understand something of Prana.

THE MENTAL PRINCIPLES.

The Western reader who has studied the writings of some of the recent Western psychologists will recognize in the Instinctive Mind certain attributes of the so-called "subjective" or "subconscious" minds spoken of so frequently by the said writers. These writers discovered in man these characteristics, as well as certain higher phases of the mind (coming from the Spiritual Mind), and without stopping to investigate further, they advanced a "new" theory that man is possessed of two minds, *i.e.*, the "objective" and "subjective," or as some have termed them, the "conscious and "subconscious." This was all very well so far as it went, but these investigators set the "conscious" mind aside and bundled all the rest into their "subconscious" or "subjective" mind, ignoring the fact that they were mixing the highest and lowest qualities of mind and putting them in the same class, and leaving the middle quality by itself. The "subjective mind" and the "subconscious" theories are very confusing, as the student finds grouped together the most sublime flashes of genius and the silliest nothings of the man of low development, the mind of the latter being almost altogether "subjective."

To those who have read up on these theories, we would say that such reading will materially help them to understand the three mental principles of man, if they will remember that the "conscious" or "objective" mind corresponds very nearly with the "Intellect" principle in the Yogi philosophy; and that the lowest portions of the "subjective" or "subconscious" mind are what the Yogis term the "Instinctive Mind" principle; while the higher and sublime qualities, which the Western writers have noticed and have grouped with the lower qualities in forming their "subjective mind" and "subconscious mind" theories, is the "Spiritual Mind" principle of the Yogis, with the difference that the "Spiritual Mind" has additional properties and qualities of which these Western theorists have never dreamed. As we touch upon each of these three mental principles, you will see the points of resemblance and the points of difference between the Yogi teachings and the Western theories.

We wish it distinctly understood, however, that we do not desire to detract from the praise justly earned by these Western investigators; in fact, the Yogis owe them a debt of gratitude for preparing the Western mind for the fuller teachings. The student who has read the works of the writers referred to will find it very much easier to grasp the idea of the three mental principles in man than if he had never heard of any division in the functioning of the mind of man. Our principal reason for calling attention to the mistake of the Western dual-mind theories was that to the mind of the Yogi it is painful to see that which he knows to be the highest manifestation of mind, that which is the seat of inspiration and flashes of genius, that which touches the pure Spirit (the Spiritual Mind), which is just beginning to awaken in men of development and growth—confused and confounded with and placed in the same class with the lowest mental principle (the Instinctive Mind) which, while most necessary and useful to man, under the direction of his higher principle is still something which is common to the most undeveloped man, even to the lower form of the animal kingdom—yea, even to the plant life. We trust that the student will free his mind of preconceived ideas on this important subject, and will listen to what we say before forming his final opinion. In our next lesson, we will go into detail regarding each of the three Mental Principles.

THE SECOND LESSON.

THE MENTAL PRINCIPLES.

IN our First Lesson we called your attention briefly to the three lower principles of man—*i.e.,* (1) the physical body; (2) the astral body; (3) Prana, or vital force. We also led up to the subject of the mental principles, which form the fourth, fifth, and sixth, respectively, of the seven principles of man.

For convenience' sake, we will again enumerate the four higher principles:

(7) Spirit.

(6) Spiritual mind.

(5) Intellect.

(4) Instinctive mind.

This terminology is more or less unsatisfactory, but we adopt it in preference to the Sanscrit terms which prove so puzzling and elusive to the average Western student.

The three lower principles are the most material, and the atoms of which they are composed are, of course, indestructible, and go on forever in countless forms and aspects; but these principles, so far as the ego is concerned, are things merely to be used in connection with a particular earth-life, just as man uses clothing, heat, electricity, etc., and they form no part of his higher nature.

The four higher principles, on the contrary, go to make up the thinking part of man—the intelligent part, so to speak. Even the lowest of the four—the instinctive mind, goes to form the higher part of the man.

Those who have not considered the subject at all are apt to regard as absurd the suggestion that the mind of man functions on more than one plane. Students of psychology, however, have long recognized the varying phases of mentation, and many theories have been advanced to account for the same. Such students will find that the Yogi philosophy alone gives the key to the mystery. Those who have studied the dual-mind theories of certain Western writers will also find it easier to conceive of more than one plane of mentality.

At first sight it would seem that the conscious, reasoning part of man's mind did the most work—if, indeed, not all of it. But a little reflection will show us that the conscious, reasoning work of the mind is but a small fraction of its task. Man's mind functions on three planes of effort, each plane shading imperceptibly into the planes on either side of it—the one next higher or the one next lower. The student may think of the matter either as one mind functioning along three lines, or as three minds shading into each other; both views have more or less of the truth in them; the real truth is too complex to be considered in detail in an elementary lesson. The principal thing is to get the idea fixed in the mind—to form mental pegs upon which to hang future information. We will touch briefly upon the several "minds," or planes of mental effort, beginning with the lowest, the instinctive mind.

(4) *The Instinctive Mind.*

This plane of mentation we share in connection with the lower animals, in, at least, its lower forms. It is the first plane of mentation reached in the scale of evolution. Its lowest phases are along lines in which consciousness is scarcely evident, and it extends from this lowly place in the scale until it manifests a very high degree of consciousness in comparison with its lowest phases; in fact, when it begins to shade into the fifth principle, it is difficult to distinguish it from the lowest forms of the latter.

The first dawn of the instinctive mind may be seen even in the mineral kingdom, more particularly in crystals, etc. Then in the plant kingdom it grows more distinct and higher in the scale, some of the higher families of plants showing even a rudimentary form of consciousness. Then in the world of the lower animals are seen increasing manifestations of the instinctive mind, from the almost plant-

like intelligence of the lower forms until we reach a
degree almost equal to that of the lowest form of
human life. Then, among men, we see it shading
gradually into the fifth principle, the intellect, until
in the highest form of man to-day we see the fifth
principle, intellect, in control to a certain extent,
and subordinating the fourth principle to it, either
wisely or unwisely. But, remember this, that even
the highest form of man carries about with him the
fourth principle, the instinctive mind, and in varying degrees uses it, or is used by it. The instinctive
mind is most useful to man in this stage of his
development—he could not exist as a physical being
without it, in fact—and he may make a most valuable servant of it if he understands it; but woe to
him if he allows it to remain in control or to usurp
prerogatives belonging to its higher brother. Now,
right here we must call your attention to the fact
that man is still a growing creature—he is not a finished product by any means. He has reached his
present stage of growth after a toilsome journey;
but it is merely sunrise yet, and the full day is far
off. The fifth principle, the intellect, has unfolded
to a certain degree, particularly in the more advanced men of to-day, but the unfoldment is merely
beginning with many. Many men are but little
more than animals, and their minds function almost
entirely upon the instinctive plane. And all men of
to-day, with the exceptions of a few very highly de-

veloped individuals, have need to be on guard lest the instinctive mind does not occasionally unduly assert its power over them, when they are off their guard.

The lowest phase of the work of the instinctive mind is akin to the same work manifesting in the plant kingdom. The work of our bodies is performed by this part of the mind. The constant work of repair, replacement, change, digestion, assimilation, elimination, etc., is being performed by this part of the mind, all below the plane of consciousness. The wondrous work of the body, in health and sickness, is faithfully carried on by this part of our minds, all without our conscious knowledge. The intelligent work of every organ, part, and cell of the body is under the superintendence of this part of the mind. Read in "Science of Breath" of the marvelous process of the circulation of the blood, its purification, etc., and realize, faintly, what a wonderful work is even this lowest phase of the instinctive mind. We will show more of its workings in our forthcoming work "Hatha Yoga," but any school physiology will give you a clear idea of what it does, although its writer does not tell the cause behind it. This part of the work of the instinctive mind is well performed in the lower animals, plants, and in man, until the latter begins to unfold a little intellect, when he often begins to meddle with the work properly belonging to this plane of the mind, and sends to it adverse suggestions, fear thoughts, etc. However, this trouble is but temporary, as, when the intellect unfolds a little farther, it sees the error into which it has fallen and proceeds to rectify the trouble and to prevent its recurrence.

But this is only a part of the province of the instinctive mind. As the animal progressed along the scale of evolution, certain things became necessary for its protection and well-being. It could not reason on these things, so that wonderful intelligence dwelling, subconsciously, in the instinctive mind unfolded until it was able to grasp the situation and meet it. It aroused the "fighting instinct" in the brute for its preservation, and this action of the instinctive mind, very good for its purpose and essential to the preservation of the life of the animal, is still with us and occasionally projects itself into our mentality with a surprising degree of strength. There is a great deal of the old animal fighting spirit in us yet, although we have managed to control it and to hold it in restraint, thanks to the light obtained from our unfolding higher faculties. The instinctive mind also taught the animal how to build its nests, how to migrate before approaching winter, how to hibernate, and thousands of other things well known to students of natural history. And it teaches us how to do the many things which we perform instinctively, as it also assumes tasks which we learn how to perform by means of our intellect, and which we pass on to the instinctive mind, which afterward performs them automatically or nearly so. It is astonishing how many of our daily tasks are performed under the direction of our instinctive mind, subject merely to a casual supervision of the Intellect. When we learn to do things "by heart," we have really mastered them on the intellectual plane, and then passed them on to the instinctive plane of mentation. The woman with her sewing-machine, the man who runs his engine, the painter with his brush, all find the instinctive mind a good friend, in fact the intellect would soon tire if it had these every-day tasks to perform. Note the difference between learning to do a thing, and then doing it after it has been learned. These manifestations of the instinctive mind are of course among its higher phases, and are due largely to its contact with and blending with the unfolding intellect.

The instinctive mind is also the "habit" mind. The intellect (either that of the owner of the instinctive mind, or of some other man) passes on ideas to it, which it afterward faithfully carries out to the letter, unless corrected or given better instructions, or worse ones, by the intellect of some one.

The instinctive mind is a queer storehouse. It is full of things received from a variety of sources. It contains many things which it has received through heredity; other things which have unfolded within it, the seeds of which were sown at the time of the primal impulse which started life along the path; other things which it has received from the intellect, including suggestions from others, as well as thought-waves sent out from the minds of others, which have taken lodgment within its corridors. All sorts of foolishness as well as wisdom is there. We will deal with this phase of the subject in future lessons, under the head of Suggestion and Auto-Suggestion, Thought Power, etc.

Instinctive mind manifests varying degrees of consciousness, varying from almost absolute subconsciousness to the simple consciousness of the highest of the lower animals and the lower forms of man. Self-consciousness comes to man with the unfoldment of the intellect, and will be spoken of in its proper place. Cosmic or universal consciousness comes with the unfoldment of the spiritual mind and will be touched upon later on. This gradual growth of consciousness is a most interesting and important branch of the subject before us, and will be referred to, and spoken of, at different points in this course.

Before we pass on to the next principle, we must call your attention to the fact that the instinctive mind is the seat of the appetites, passions, desires, instincts, sensations, feelings, and emotions of the lower order, manifested in man as well as in the lower animals. There are of course higher ideas, emotions, aspirations, and desires, reaching the advanced man from the unfolding spiritual mind, but the animal desires, and the ordinary feelings, emotions, etc., belong to the instinctive mind. All the "feelings" belonging to our passional and emotional nature belong to this plane. All animal desires, such as hunger and thirst, sexual desires (on the physical plane) ; all passions, such as physical love, hatred, envy, malice, jealousy, revenge, are a part of it. The desire for the physical (unless as a means of reaching higher things), the longing for the material, all belong to this plane. The "lust of the flesh, the lust of the eyes, the pride of life," are on this plane. This principle is the most material of the three mental principles, and is the one which is apt to bind us the closest to the earth and earthly things. Remember, that we are not condemning material or "earthly" things—they are all right in their place; but man in his unfoldment grows to see these things as only a means to an end—only a step in the spiritual evolution. And with clearer vision he ceases to be bound too tightly to the material side of life, and, instead of regarding it as the end and aim of all things, sees that it is, at the best, only a means to a higher end.

Many of the "brute" instincts are still with us, and are much in evidence in undeveloped people. Occultists learn to curb and control these lower instincts, and to subordinate them to the higher mental ideals which open up to them. Be not discouraged, dear student, if you find much of the animal still within you. It is no sign of "badness," or evil; in fact the recognition of it by one is a sign that his unfoldment has begun, for, before, the same thing was there and not recognized for what it is, whereas now it is both seen and recognized. Knowledge is power; learn to know the remnants of the brute nature within you and become a tamer of wild beasts. The higher principles will always obtain the mastery, but patience, perseverance, and faith are required for the task. These "brute" things were all right in their time—the animal had need of them— they were "good" for the purpose intended, but now that man is reaching higher points on the path, he sees clearer and learns to subordinate the lower parts of himself to the higher. The lower instincts were not implanted in your nature by "the devil"; you came by them honestly. They came in the process of evolution as a proper and right thing, but have been largely outgrown and can now be left behind. So do not fear these inheritances from the past; you can put them aside or subordinate them to higher things as you journey along the path. Do not despise them, though you tread them under foot — they are the steps upon which you have reached your present high estate, and upon which you will attain still greater heights.

(5) *The Intellect.*

We now reach the mental principle which distin-

guishes man from the brute. The first four principles man shares in common with the lower forms of
life, but when the fifth principle begins to unfold
he has reached an important stage of the journey
along the path of attainment. He feels his manhood manifesting within him.

Now, remember, that there is no violent change
or marked transition from the consciousness of the
fourth principle into that of the fifth. As we have
before explained, these principles shade into each
other, and blend as do the colors of the spectrum.
As intellect unfolds, it illuminates faintly the fourth
principle, and endows instinctive life with reason.
Simple consciousness shades into self-consciousness.
Before the fifth principle dawns fairly, the creature
having the four principles well developed has passions but no reason; emotions but not intellect; desires but no rationalized will. It is the subject
awaiting the monarch, the sleeper awaiting the
magic touch of the one who has been sent to awaken
him from the enchanter's deep sleep. It is the
brute awaiting the coming of that which will trans-
form it into a man.

In some of the lower animals, the fourth principle has attracted to itself the lowest shading of the
fifth principle, and the animal manifests signs of a
faint reasoning. On the other hand, in some of the
lower forms of man—the Bushman, for example—
the fourth principle has scarcely been perceptibly

colored by the incoming fifth principle, and the
"man" is scarcely more than a brute, in fact is more
of a brute, mentally, than some of the higher do-
mesticated animals, who, having been for many
generations in close companionship with man, have
been colored by his mental emanations.

The first sign of the real unfoldment of the fifth
principle, intellect, is the dawning of self-consciousness. In order more fully to understand this, let us
consider what consciousness really is.

Among the lower animals there is very little of
that which we call consciousness. The consciousness of the lower animal forms is but little more
than mere sensation. Life in the early stages is
almost automatic. The mentation is almost entirely
along subconscious lines, and the mentation itself is
only that which is concerned with the physical life
of the animal—the satisfaction of its primitive wants.
After a bit, this primitive consciousness developed
into what psychologists term simple consciousness.
Simple consciousness is an "awareness" of outside
things—a perception and recognition of things other
than the inner self. The conscious attention is
turned outward. The animal or low order of man,
cannot think of his hopes and fears, his aspirations,
his plans, his thoughts, and then compare them
with the like thoughts of others of his kind. He
cannot turn his gaze inward and speculate upon
abstract things. He simply takes things for granted

and asks no questions. He does not attempt to find solutions for questions within himself, for he is not aware that such questions exist.

With the advent of self-consciousness man begins to form a conception of the "I." He begins to compare himself with others and to reason about it. He takes mental stock, and draws conclusions from what he finds in his mind. He begins to think for himself, to analyze, classify, separate, deduce, etc. As he progresses he begins to think out things for himself, and passes along new and fresh suggestions to his instinctive mind. He begins to rely upon his own mind, rather than blindly accepting that which emanates from the mind of others. He begins to create for himself, and is no longer a mere mental automaton.

And from a mere glimmering of conscious intelligence there has grown the highest intelligence of to-day. A modern writer forcibly expresses the growth in the following words: "For some hundreds of years, upon the general plane of self-consciousness, an ascent, to the human eye gradually, but from the point of view of cosmic evolution rapid, has been made. In a race, large-brained, walking erect, gregarious, brutal, but king of all other brutes, man in appearance but not in fact, was from the highest simple-consciousness born the basic human faculty self-consciousness, and its twin, language. From these and what went with these, through suffering, toil, and war; through bestiality, savagery, barbarism; through slavery, greed, effort; through conquests infinite, through defeats overwhelming, through struggle unending; through ages of aimless semi-brutal existence; through subsistence on berries and roots; through the use of the casually found stone or stick; through life in deep forests, with nuts and seeds, and on the shores of waters with mollusks, crustaceans, and fish for food; through that greatest, perhaps, of human victories, the domestication and subjugation of fire; through the invention and art of bow and arrow; through the taming of animals and the breaking of them to labor; through the long learning which led to the cultivation of the soil; through the adobe brick and the building of houses therefrom; through the smelting of metals and the slow birth of the arts which rest upon these; through the slow making of alphabets and the evolution of the written word; in short, through thousands of centuries of human life, of human aspiration, of human growth, sprang the world of men and women as it stands before us and within us to-day with all its achievements and possessions."

Self-consciousness is a thing easy to comprehend, but difficult to define. One writer has expressed it well when he says that without self-consciousness a creature may *know;* but only by the aid of self-consciousness is it possible for him to *know that he knows.*

And with this unfoldment of the intellect came the beginnings of all the wonderful achievements of the human mind of to-day. But great as are these achievements, these are as nothing to what is yet before the race. From victory on to victory will the intellect progress. In its unfoldment, as it begins to receive more and more light from the next highest principle, the spiritual mind, it will achieve things as yet undreamed of. And yet, poor mortal, remember, intellect is third from the highest in the scale on the principles of man. There are two principles as much higher than intellect, as intellect is higher than the principle below—instinctive mind. Do not make a God of intellect; do not allow the pride of intellect to blind you.

The importance of the awakening of self-consciousness may be more clearly recognized when we tell you that the occult doctrine is that once the self-consciousness is awakened into being, once the "I" has been felt and recognized, the real awakened life of the soul begins. We do not refer to the life that comes after the spiritual awakening—that is a still higher stage—but to the mental awakening of the soul to the "I" consciousness. This is the stage where the baby ego first begins its waking existence. Previous to that time it has slumbered on, alive but not conscious of itself, and now the time of labor pains and birth is at hand. The soul has to meet new conditions, and has many an obstacle to overcome before it reaches spiritual manhood. Many experiences will it undergo, many trials will it be forced to meet; but still the progress is on and on and on.

At times there may be setbacks, and it may even seem to retrograde, but such obstacles are soon surmounted and the soul takes up its journey again. There is no real going backward on the path, and slow as the progress may seem, each of us is moving steadily forward.

We had hoped to be able to reach the subject of the sixth principle, spiritual mind, in this lesson, but we see that we have not sufficient space at our disposal, so we must defer that most interesting subject, as well as that of the seventh principle, spirit, until the next lesson. We are aware that our students are eager to press forward, and we are wasting as little time as possible on the way; but there are certain fundamental truths which must be clearly understood before we dare take another step.

There are a number of lessons to be drawn from the subjects of the instinctive mind and the intellect, and this is as good a place as any in which to consider them.

One of these lessons is that the awakening of intellect does not necessarily make the creature a better being, in the sense of being "good." While it is true that an unfolding principle or faculty will give an upward tendency to man, it is equally true that some men are so closely wrapped in the folds of the animal sheath—so steeped in the material side of things—that the awakened intellect only tends to give them increased powers to gratify their low desires and inclinations. Man, if he chooses, may excel the beasts in bestiality—he may descend to depths of which the beast would never have thought. The beast is governed solely by instinct, and his actions, so prompted, are perfectly natural and proper, and the animal is not blamed for following the impulses of its nature. But man, in whom intellect has unfolded, knows that it is contrary to his highest nature to descend to the level of the beasts— yea, lower by far. He adds to the brute desires the cunning and intelligence which have come to him, and deliberately prostitutes his higher principle to the task of carrying out the magnified animal propensities. Very few animals abuse their desires—it is left for some men to do so. The higher the degree of intellect unfolded in a man, the greater the depths of low passions, appetites, and desires possible to him. He actually creates new brute desires, or rather, builds edifices of his own upon the brute foundations. It is unnecessary for us to state that all occultists know that such a course will bring certain consequences in its train, which will result in the soul having to spend many weary years in retracing its steps over the backward road it has trodden. Its progress has been retarded, and it will be com-

pelled to retravel the road to freedom, in common
with the beast-like natures of undeveloped creatures
whose proper state of the journey it is, having an
additional burden in the shape of the horror of consciousness of its surroundings, whereas its companions have no such consciousness and consequently
suffer not. If you can imagine a civilized, refined
man having to live among Australian Bushmen for
many years, with a full recollection of what he has
lost, you may form a faint idea of the fate in store
for one who deliberately sinks his high powers to
the accomplishment of low ends and desires. But
even for such a soul there is escape—in time.

Let your higher nature be on guard and refuse to
be drawn back into the brute life which has been
passed through. Keep your gaze upward, and let
your motto be: "Forward." The brute nature may
exert a pull downward, but the spiritual mind will
give you a helping hand, and will sustain you if you
but trust to it. The intellect is between the two,
and may be influenced by either or both. Take
your choice, oh, struggling soul. Your help is within you; look to it, and refuse to be dragged back
into the mire of the animal mind. Manifest the "I"
within you and be strong. You are an immortal
soul, and are moving on and on and on to still
greater things. Peace be yours.

THE THIRD LESSON.

THE SPIRITUAL PRINCIPLES.

In our Second Lesson we gave you a brief outline of the Fourth and Fifth Principles of Man, *i.e.*, (4) Instinctive Mind, and (5) Intellect. As we have told you before, man has passed through the Fourth Principle stage to its extreme, and has now passed on to a consciousness of the Fifth Principle, Intellect. Some of us have developed the Intellectual stage to a considerable extent (although we have practically conquered but a few square miles of the new territory of the mind, and there is still a great task before us), while other men seem to have a consciousness almost altogether within the borders of the Instinctive Mind, and have only a glimmering of Intellect. Not only is this true of the savage races, but many, very many of so-called "civilized" people have not learned to do their own thinking, and seem willing to allow others to do their thinking for them, they following certain leaders with the stupid habit of the sheep. But still the race is progressing, slowly but surely, and many are thinking now who never thought before—a greater num-

37

ber are refusing to take their thinking second-hand, and are insisting upon knowing for themselves.

When we consider that there are many men in whom the Fifth Principle, the Intellect, has scarcely unfolded, and that the race in general has taken but a few steps into the land of the Intellect, we begin to realize how difficult it is for any of us except the man or woman of exceptional spiritual unfoldment to comprehend even faintly the still higher Principles. It is something like a man born blind trying to comprehend light; or one born deaf endeavoring to form a mental concept of sound. One can only form an idea of something akin to his experiences. A man who has never tasted anything sweet cannot form an idea of sugar. Without experience or consciousness of a thing, our minds are unable to form a concept.

But nearly all of us who have been attracted to these lessons or who have attracted these lessons to us, have had experiences which will enable us to comprehend something of the Sixth Principle—have had glimmerings of consciousness which help us to understand something of the Spiritual Mind. A tendency toward the occult—the hunger of the soul for more light—are indications that the Sixth Principle, Spiritual Mind, is beginning to shade into our consciousness, and, although it may be ages before we awaken into full Spiritual Consciousness, we are still being influenced and helped by it. This spiritual unrest often causes us great discomfort, until we find ourselves on the right road to knowledge, and even thereafter we feel more or less unsatisfied by the few crumbs that drop to us from the table of Knowledge. But despair not, seekers after the Truth; these pains are but the travail of spiritual birth—great things are before you—take courage and fear not.

Toward the end of this lesson we will speak of the process of "Illumination" or Spiritual Consciousness, which has come, or is coming, to many of us, and what we have to say may throw light upon many experiences which have come to you, and for which you have heretofore had no explanation.

We will now take up the subject of the Sixth Principle, Spiritual Mind, which will be more or less plain to those who have had glimmerings of consciousness from this plane of the soul, but which will be full of "hard sayings" and "dark corners" to those who have not as yet reached this stage of unfoldment. The Seventh Principle, The Spirit, however, is beyond the comprehension of any except the few enlightened and highly developed souls, in and out of the body, who are as far above the ordinary man as the average enlightened man is above the Bushman. We can but pass on to you enough to give you a general intellectual idea of what is meant by "Spirit"—the consciousness of it is still far beyond the race in its present stage. It is well, however, to know of the existence of Spirit, as it helps us to understand something of the Spiritual Mind, which is Spirit's means of communication with the Intellectual consciousness. The comprehension of Spiritual Mind, however, opens up such a wonderful world of thought that we are satisfied to leave the understanding of Spirit until such time as we will grow into a consciousness of it.

(6) *The Spiritual Mind.*

The Sixth Principle, Spiritual Mind, has been styled by some writers "The Superconscious Mind," which term is a fairly good one, as it distinguishes between the lower Subconscious Mind or Instinctive Mind, the Conscious Mind or Intellect, and itself, which latter, while outside of the realm of ordinary human consciousness, is still a very different thing from the lower or Instinctive Mind.

While the actual existence of the Spiritual Mind has been made manifest to but a limited number of the human race, there are many who are becoming conscious of a higher "Something Within," which leads them up to higher and nobler thoughts, desires, aspirations, and deeds. And there is a still greater number who receive a faint glimmering of the light of the Spirit, and, though they know it not, are more or less influenced by it. In fact, the entire race receives some of its beneficent rays, although in some cases the light is so bedimmed by the dense material obstacles surrounding the man that his spiritual twilight is almost akin to the blackness of night. But man is ever unfolding, discarding sheath after sheath, and is slowly coming home. The light will eventually shine full upon all.

All that we consider good, noble, and great in the human mind emanates from the Spiritual Mind and is gradually unfolded into the ordinary consciousness. Some Eastern writers prefer the term "projected" as more correctly indicating the process whereby the ray of light is sent into the consciousness of the man who has not yet reached the superhuman stage of full Spiritual Consciousness. All that has come to man, in his evolution, which tends toward nobility, true religious feeling, kindness, humanity, justice, unselfish love, mercy, sympathy, etc., has come to him through his slowly unfolding Spiritual Mind. His love of God and his love of Man has come to him in this way. As the unfoldment goes on, his idea of Justice enlarges; he has more Compassion; his feeling of Human Brotherhood increases; his idea of Love grows; and he increases in all the qualities which men of all creeds pronounce "good," and which may all be summed up as the practical attempt to live out the teachings of that great spiritual Master, when He enunciated that great truth (well understood by the occultists of all creeds, but so little understood by many who claim to be followers of Him), saying: "And thou shalt love the Lord, thy God, with all thy heart, and with all thy soul, and with all thy mind, and with all thy strength," and "Thou shalt love thy neighbor as thyself."

As man's Spiritual Consciousness begins to unfold, he begins to have an abiding sense of the reality of the existence of the Supreme Power, and, growing along with it, he finds the sense of Human Brotherhood — of human relationship — gradually coming into consciousness. He does not get these things from his Instinctive Mind, nor does his Intellect make him *feel* them. Spiritual Mind does not run contrary to Intellect — it simply goes beyond Intellect. It passes down to the Intellect certain truths which it finds in its own regions of the mind, and Intellect reasons about them. But they do not originate with Intellect. Intellect is cold—Spiritual Consciousness is warm and alive with high feeling.

Man's growth toward a better and fuller idea of the Divine Power does not come from Intellect, although the latter reasons upon the impressions received and tries to form them into systems, creeds, cults, etc. Nor does the Intellect give us our growing sense of the relationship between man and man —the Brotherhood of Man. Let us tell you why man is kinder to his kind and to forms of life below him than ever before. It is not alone because the Intellect teaches him the value of kindness and love, for man does not become kind or loving by cold reasoning. On the contrary, he becomes kind and loving because there arise within him certain impulses and desires coming from some unknown place, which render it impossible for him to be otherwise without suffering discomfort and pain. These impulses are as real as other desires and impulses, and as man develops these impulses become more numerous and much stronger. Look at the world of a few hundred years ago, and look at it to-day, and see how much kinder and more loving we are than in those days. But do not boast of it, for we will seem as mere savages to those who follow us and who will wonder at our inhumanity to our brother-man from their point of view.

As man unfolds spiritually he feels his relationship to all mankind, and he begins to love his fellow-man more and more. It hurts him to see others suffering, and when it hurts him enough he tries to do something to remedy it. As time goes on and man develops, the terrible suffering which many human beings undergo to-day will be impossible, for the reason that the unfolding Spiritual Consciousness of the race will make the pain felt so severely by all that the race will not be able to stand it, and they will insist upon matters being remedied. From the inner recesses of the soul comes a protest against the following of the lower animal nature, and, although we may put it aside for a time, it will become more and more persistent, until we are forced to heed it. The old story of each person having two advisors, one at each ear, one whispering to him to follow the higher teachings and the other tempting him to pursue the lower path, is shown to be practically true by the occult teaching regarding the three mental principles. The Intellect represents the "I" consciousness of the average person. This "I" has on one side the Instinctive Mind sending him to the old desires of the former self—the impulses of the less developed life of the animal or lower man, which desires were all very well in lower stages of development, but which are unworthy of the growing man. On the other side is the Spiritual Mind, sending its unfolding impulses into the Intellect, and endeavoring to draw the consciousness up to itself—to aid in the man's unfoldment and development, and to cause him to master and control his lower nature.

The struggle between the higher and lower natures has been noticed by all careful observers of the human mind and character, and many have been the theories advanced to account for it. In former times it was taught that man was being tempted by the devil on the one hand, and helped by a guardian angel on the other. But the truth is known to all occultists that the struggle is between the two elements of man's nature, not exactly warring, but each following its own line of effort, and the "I" being torn and bruised in its efforts to adjust itself.

The Ego is in a transition stage of consciousness, and the struggle is quite painful at times, but the growing man in time rises above the attraction of the lower nature, and dawning Spiritual Consciousness enables him to understand the true state of affairs, and aids him in asserting his mastery over the lower self and in assuming a positive attitude toward it, while at the same time he opens himself up to the light from the Spiritual Mind and holds himself in a negative attitude toward it, resisting not its power.

The Spiritual Mind is also the source of the "inspiration" which certain poets, painters, sculptors, writers, preachers, orators, and others have received in all times and which they receive to-day. This is the source from which the seer obtains his vision— the prophet his foresight. Many have concentrated themselves upon high ideals in their work, and have received rare knowledge from this source, and have attributed it to beings of another world — from angels, spirits, from God Himself; but all came from within—is was the voice of their Higher Self speaking to them. We do not mean to say that no communications come to man from other intelligences —far from this, we *know* that higher intelligences do often communicate with man through the channel of his Spiritual Mind—but much that man has attributed to outside intelligences has really come from himself. And man, by the development of his

Spiritual Consciousness, may bring himself into a high relationship and contact with this higher part of his nature, and may thus become possessed of a knowledge of which the Intellect has not dared dream.

Certain high psychic powers are also open to man in this way, but such powers are rarely obtained by one until he has risen above the attractions of the lower part of his nature, for unless this were so man might use these high gifts for base purposes. It is only when man ceases to care for power for his personal use that power comes. Such is the Law.

When man learns of the existence of his Spiritual mind and begins to recognize its promptings and leadings, he strengthens his bond of communication with it, and consequently receives light of a greater brilliancy. When we learn to trust the Spirit, it responds by sending us more frequent flashes of illumination and enlightenment. As one unfolds in Spiritual Consciousness he relies more upon this Inner Voice, and is able more readily to distinguish it from impulses from the lower planes of the mind. He learns to follow Spirit's leadings and to allow it to lend him a guiding hand. Many of us have learned to know the reality of being "led by the Spirit." To those who have experienced this leading we need not say more, for they will recognize just what we mean. Those who have not as yet experienced it must wait until the time comes for them, for we cannot describe it, as there are no words to speak of these things which are beyond words.

Toward the close of this lesson we will give a brief outline of some of the phases of "Illumination" or awakening of Spiritual Consciousness, which has come to some of us and will come to all in this or future phases of their unfoldment. We must hasten on to a brief consideration of that which can only be faintly understood by any of us— the Seventh Principle—Spirit.

(7) *Spirit.*

How shall we approach this subject, which even the most advanced minds in the flesh to-day can but faintly comprehend? How can the finite express or comprehend the infinite? Spirit, man's Seventh Principle, is the Divine Spark—our most precious inheritance from the Divine Power—a ray from the Central Sun—the Real Self. Words cannot express it. Our minds fail to grasp it. It is the soul of the Soul. To understand it we must understand God, for Spirit is a drop from the Spirit Ocean—a grain of sand from the shores of the Infinite—a particle of the Sacred Flame. It is that something within us which is the cause of our evolution through all the weary ages. It was the first to be, and yet it will be the last to appear in full consciousness. When man arrives at a full consciousness of Spirit, he will be so much higher than man that such a being is at present inconceivable to the Intellect. Confined in many sheaths of matter, it has waited through the long and weary ages for even a faint recognition, and is content to wait for ages more until it is fully brought into consciousness. Man will ascend many steps of development—from man to archangel—before Spirit will fully claim its own. The Spirit is that within man which closest approaches the Center—is nearest to God. It is only in an occasional precious moment that we are aware of the existence of Spirit within us, and in such moments we are conscious of coming into the awful presence of the Unknown. These moments may come when one is engaged in deep religious thought—while reading a poem bearing a precious message from soul to soul —in some hour of affliction when all human aid has failed us and when human words seem but mockery —in a moment when all seems lost and we feel the necessity of a direct word from a being higher than ourselves. When these moments come they leave with us a peace which never afterward entirely escapes us, and we are ever after changed beings. In the moment of Illumination or the dawn of Spiritual Consciousness we also feel the real presence of the Spirit. In these moments we become conscious of our relationship with and connection with the Center of Life. Through the medium of the Spirit God reveals Himself to Man.

We cannot dwell longer on this subject—it over-powers one, and mere words seem too weak for use in connection with it. Those who have felt the im-pulses of the Spiritual Mind have been made faintly conscious of the abiding sense of the Spirit, although they cannot grasp its full significance. And those who have not experienced these things would not understand us if we wrote volumes of our imperfect and undeveloped conceptions of the subject. So we will pass on, trusting that we have awakened in your minds at least a faint desire to be brought into a closer communion and contact with this, the high-est part of Self—Self itself. The Peace of the Spirit abide with you.

Illumination or Spiritual Consciousness.

With many, Spiritual Mind unfolds gradually and slowly, and, while one may feel a steady increase of spiritual knowledge and consciousness, he may not have experienced any marked and startling change. Others have had moments of what is known as "Illumination," when they seemed lifted almost out of their normal state, and where they seemed to pass into a higher plane of consciousness or being, which left them more advanced than ever before, although they could not carry back into conscious-ness a clear recollection of what they had experi-enced while in the exalted state of mind. These experiences have come to many persons, in different forms and degrees, of all forms of religious beliefs, and have been generally associated with some feature of the particular religious belief entertained by the person experiencing the illumination. But advanced occultists recognize all of these experiences as differing forms of one and the same thing— the dawning of the Spiritual Consciousness—the unfoldment of the Spiritual Mind. Some writers have styled this experience "Cosmic Consciousness," which is a very appropriate name, as the illumination, at least in its higher forms, brings one in touch with the whole of Life, making him feel a sense of kinship with all Life, high or low, great or small, "good" or "bad."

These experiences, of course, vary materially according to the degree of unfoldment of the individual, his previous training, his temperament, etc., but certain characteristics are common to all. The most common feeling is that of possessing almost complete knowledge of all things—almost Omniscience. This feeling exists only for a moment, and leaves one at first in an agony of regret over what he has seen and lost. Another feeling commonly experienced is that of a certainty of immortality—a sense of actual *being,* and the certainty of having always been, and of being destined to always be. Another feeling is the total slipping away of all fear and the acquirement of a feeling of certainty, trust, and confidence, which is beyond the comprehension of those who have never experienced it. Then a feeling of love sweeps over one—a love which takes in all Life, from those near to one in the flesh to those at the farthest parts of the universe—from those whom we hold as pure and holy to those whom the world regards as vile, wicked, and utterly unworthy. All feelings of self-righteousness and condemnation seem to slip away, and one's love, like the light of the sun, falls upon all alike, irrespective of their degree of development or "goodness."

To some these experiences have come as a deep, reverent mood or feeling, which took complete possession of them for a few moments or longer, while others have seemed in a dream and have become conscious of a spiritual uplifting accompanied by a sensation of being surrounded by a brilliant and all-pervading light or glow. To some certain truths have become manifest in the shape of symbols, the true meaning of which did not become apparent until, perhaps, long afterward.

These experiences, when they have come to one, have left him in a new state of mind, and he has never been the same man afterward. Although the keenness of the recollection has worn off, there remains a certain memory which long afterward proves a source of comfort and strength to him, especially when he feels faint of faith and is shaken like a reed by the winds of conflicting opinions and speculations of the Intellect. The memory of such an ex-

perience is a source of renewed strength—a haven of
refuge to which the weary soul flies for shelter from
the outside world, which understands it not.

These experiences are usually also accompanied
with a sense of intense joy; in fact, the word and
thought "Joy" seems to be uppermost in the mind
at the time. But it is a joy not of ordinary experience—it is something which cannot be dreamed of
until after one has experienced it—it is a joy the
recollection of which will cause the blood to tingle
and the heart to throb whenever the mind reverts to
the experience. As we have already said, there also
comes a sense of a "knowing" of all things—an intellectual illumination impossible to describe.

From the writings of the ancient philosophers of
all races, from the songs of the great poets of all
peoples, from the preachings of the prophets of all
religions and times we can gather traces of this
illumination which has come to them—this unfoldment of the Spiritual Consciousness. We have not
the space to enumerate these numerous instances.
One has told of it in one way, the other in another;
but all tell practically the same story. All who have
experienced this illumination, even in a faint degree, recognize the like experience in the tale, song,
or preaching of another, though centuries may roll
between them. It is the song of the Soul, which
when once heard is never forgotten. Though it be
sounded by the crude instrument of the semibar-

barous races or the finished instrument of the talented musician of to-day, its strains are plainly recognized. From Old Egypt comes the song—from India in all ages—from Ancient Greece and Rome— from the early Christian saint—from the Quaker Friend—from the Catholic monasteries—from the Mohammedan mosque—from the Chinese philosopher—from the legends of the American Indian hero-prophet—it is always the same strain, and it is swelling louder and louder, as many more are taking it up and adding their voices or the sounds of their instruments to the grand chorus.

That much-misunderstood Western poet, Walt Whitman, knew what he meant (and so do we) when he blurted out in uncouth verse his strange experiences. Read what he says—has it ever been better expressed?

"As in a swoon, one instant,
Another sun, ineffable, full dazzles me,
And all the orbs I knew, and brighter, unknown orbs,
One instant of the future land, Heaven's land."

And when he rouses himself from his ecstasy, he cries:

"I cannot be awake, for nothing looks to me as it did before,
Or else I am awake for the first time, and all before has been a mean sleep."

And we must join with him when he expresses

man's inability to describe intelligently this thing in these words:

> "When I try to tell the best I find, I cannot;
> My tongue is ineffectual on its pivots,
> My breath will not be obedient to its organs,
> I become a dumb man."

May this great joy of Illumination be yours, dear students. And it will be yours when the proper time comes. When it comes do not be dismayed, and when it leaves you do not mourn its loss—it will come again. Live on, reaching ever upward toward your Real Self and opening up yourself to its influence. Be always willing to listen to the Voice of The Silence—willing always to respond to the touch of The Unseen Hand. In the little manual, "Light on the Path," you will find many things which will now perhaps seem plainer to you.

Do not fear again, for you have with you always the Real Self, which is a spark from the Divine Flame, and which will be as a lamp to your feet to show you the way.

Peace be unto you.

THE FOURTH LESSON.

THE HUMAN AURA.

In our previous three lessons we called your attention briefly, in turn, to the Seven Principles of Man. The subject of the Constitution of Man, however, is incomplete without a reference to what occultists know as the Human Aura. This forms a most interesting part of the occult teachings, and reference to it is to be found in the occult writings and traditions of all races. Considerable misapprehension and confusion regarding the Human Aura have arisen, and the truth has been obscured by the various speculations and theories of some of the writers on the subject. This is not to be wondered at when we remember that the Aura is visible only to those of highly developed psychic power. Some possessing inferior sight, which has enabled them to see only certain of the grosser manifestations of the emanation constituting the Aura, have thought and taught that what they saw was all that could be seen; while the real truth is, that such people have seen but a part of the whole thing, the remainder being reserved for those of higher development.

Some teachers of late years have taught that the Aura was really the several principles of man, projecting beyond the space occupied by his physical body; but this is only true in the same sense that the light of the sun is a part of the sun—the rays of the electric light a part of the light—the heat radiating from a stove the heat contained within the stove—the odor of a flower the flower itself. The Aura is really an emanation of one or more of the seven principles of man—radiations sent forth from the principle itself—and not, strictly speaking, a part of the principle, except in the sense above referred to.

Each of the seven principles of which man is composed radiates energy which is visible to the developed psychic senses of certain of our race. This radiated energy is akin to the radiations known as the "X-Ray," and like them is invisible to the human eye unless aided by something which the human eye does not ordinarily possess. Some of the grosser forms of the Aura are visible to those possessing a comparatively undeveloped grade of psychic power, while the higher forms become visible only as the psychic faculties develop in power. There are but comparatively few in the flesh to-day who have ever seen the Aura emanating from the sixth principle, the Spiritual Mind. And the Aura of the seventh principle, the Spirit, is visible only to those beings far higher in the scale than the human race as we know it. The Aura emanating from the lower five principles is seen by many of us who have developed psychic power, our clearness of vision and range of sight being determined by the particular state of development we have reached.

We will try to give our students a general idea of the Human Aura and a hasty outline of that which pertains to it in this lesson, but it will readily be seen that the subject is one that could not be exhausted in a volume of considerable size. It is a difficult matter to condense information of this nature, but we trust to be able to convey a fairly clear impression of the subject to those of our students who will follow us closely.

As we have already stated, each principle radiates energy which, combining, constitutes what is known as the Human Aura. The Aura of each principle, if the other principles be removed, would occupy the same space as that filled by the Aura of all or any of the other principles. In other words, the several Auras of the different principles interpenetrate each other, and, being of different rates of vibration, do not interfere one with the other. When we speak of The Aura, we mean the entire Aura of the man, visible to one of psychic sight. When we speak of the Aura emanating from any particular principle, we distinctly refer to the principle.

The grossest form of the human Aura is, of course, that emanating from the physical body. This is sometimes spoken of as the "Health Aura," as it is a sure indication of the state of the physical health of the person from whose body it radiates. Like all other forms of the Aura, it extends from the body to a distance of two to three feet, depending upon certain circumstances which need not be mentioned at this place. Like all other forms of the Aura, it is oval or egg-shaped. (This shape common to the several manifestations of the Aura has caused some writers to refer to it as the "Auric Egg.") The physical Aura is practically colorless (or possibly almost a bluish-white, resembling the color of clear water), but possessing a peculiar feature not possessed by the other manifestations of Aura, inasmuch as to the psychic vision it appears to be "streaked" by numerous fine lines extending like stiff bristles from the body outward. In normal health and vitality these "bristles" stand out stiffly, while in cases of impaired vitality or poor health they droop like the soft hair on an animal, and in some cases present the appearance of a ruffled coat of hair, the several "hairs" standing out in all directions, tangled, twisted, and curled. This phenomenon is occasioned by the current of prana energizing the body to a greater or lesser extent, the healthy body having the normal supply of prana, while the diseased or weak body suffers from an insufficient supply. This physical Aura is seen by many having a very limited degree of psychic sight and to whom the higher forms of Aura are invisible. To the developed psychic it is sometimes difficult to distinguish, owing to its being obscured by the colors in the higher forms of Aura, the psychic, in order to observe it, being compelled to inhibit the impressions of the higher forms of Aura and to admit only the vibration of the particular form of Aura which he wishes to observe. Particles detached from the physical Aura remain around the spot or place where the person has been, and a strongly developed sense found in dogs and other animals enables them to follow up the "scent" of the person or animal they are tracking.

The Aura emanating from the second principle, or Astral Body, is, like the principle itself, of a vapor-like appearance and color, having a resemblance to steam just before it dissolves and disappears from sight. It is difficult to distinguish when it is intermingled with the other forms of Aura, but when the astral body is seen apart from the physical body its Aura may be perceived, particularly if the observer is not open to the vibrations from the principles sending forth Auras of various colors. Those of our readers who have ever seen an astral form, or what is commonly called a "ghost' of high or low degree, will probably remember having seen a cloudy egg-shape vapor surrounding the more distinct figure of the astral form. This faint, vapor-like, oval cloud was the astral Aura. It, of course, becomes visible to one to whom an astral form "materializes."

The Aura of the third principle, or Prana, is difficult to describe except to those who have seen the
"X-Ray." It looks something like a vapory cloud
of the color and appearance of an electric spark. In
fact, all manifestations of Prana resemble electric
light or sparks. Prana has a faint rosy tint when it
is in or near the body, but loses this hue as it gets a
few inches away. Persons of psychic sight see
plainly the spark-like particles of Prana being shaken
from the finger-tips of persons giving so-called "magnetic treatments" or making mesmeric passes. It
may also be seen by many persons who make no
claims of psychic sight, to whom it appears like
heated air arising from a stove or from the heated
ground, that is to say, as a colorless something pulsating and vibrating. This pranic Aura is sometimes drawn away from a healthy strong person by a
weak person who is lacking in vitality and who
draws away from the strong one that which is needed
by the weak one. In cases of this kind, the person
drawn upon without his consent will experience a
feeling of languor and lassitude after being in the
company of the person who has absorbed a share of
his vitality. In "Science of Breath," on page 61,
under the head " (2) Forming an Aura," we have
given a method whereby one may render himself
immune to this form of vampirism, conscious or unconscious. This method, while given in the book
for another purpose, is equally efficacious in this in-

stance. A stronger effect may be produced by forming a mental image of an Auric shell through which
no force can escape or no outside influence enter
without one's own consent.   One may in this way
also guard himself against infection from sources
which might seriously affect him unless so protected.
The pranic Aura is also poured out in mesmeric
passes or psychic "treatments" of the sick, but in
such cases the trained operator regulates the flow
and takes the trouble to replenish the supply of
prana within his system, which will generate and
emanate a constant flow of pranic Aura.   We need
not dwell upon these points, as they are fully described in "Science of Breath," which book will be
read with a new light by the student who reads and
thinks over what we have said about this feature of
the Human Aura.   The little book in question was
written for the general public, who, while they will
receive much benefit from it, cannot read from it
the meaning which becomes perfectly clear to the
student as he passes from stage to stage of these lessons.   The little book, simple and unpretentious as
it is, has many things hidden away in it which may
only be read by the one who is able to understand.
The student is advised to re-read the little book
from time to time and notice how many things he
finds in it which he never before discovered.

We now approach the most interesting features
concerning the Human Aura, and we think that

some of the facts to be stated in this lesson will be a revelation even to many who are perfectly familiar with the three manifestations of the Aura which we have just mentioned. Some may doubt many of the statements which will be made, but we beg to say to such people that they have the means at their disposal to develop and unfold psychic powers of a sufficient degree to see these things for themselves as thousands of others before them have done. Nothing of the occult teachings need remain hidden to any one who doubts. Every one may enter the occult world for himself—providing he pays the price of attainment, which price is not of gold or silver, but of the renunciation of the lower self and the devotion to that which is highest in man. Some, it is true, break into the psychic world without having fitted and purified themselves by the proper methods, but to such the acquired faculties are a curse rather than a blessing, and such are compelled to retrace their steps with much suffering until they enter in by the right door, the key of which is readily found by all who seek for it in the proper spirit.

To return to the higher manifestations of the Human Aura, we again call your attention to the fact that the Aura is seen by the psychic observer as a luminous cloud, nearly oval in shape, extending from two feet to three feet in all directions from the body. It does not terminate abruptly, but gradually fades into faintness until it disappears entirely. It really extends quite a distance beyond its visible point. It presents the appearance of a luminous cloud of constantly shifting colors, certain colors, however, being predominant in each person, from reasons which we will consider in a few moments. These colors originate from certain mental states of the person whom the Aura surrounds. Each thought, emotion, or feeling is manifested by a certain shade or combination of colors belonging to that particular thought, emotion, or feeling, which color or colors manifest themselves in the Aura of that particular mental principle in which the thought, emotion, or feeling naturally originates, and are of course visible to the observer studying the composite Aura of the thinker. The developed psychic may read the thoughts of a person as he can the pages of an open book, providing he understands the language of the Auric colors, which, of course, all developed occultists do, although the person who stumbles accidentally into the psychic world on rare occasions will see nothing but the reflection of wonderful colors appearing in a luminous cloud, the meaning of which is not known to him.

We think it better, before proceeding further, to give you a general idea of these Auric colors, and the thought, feeling, or emotion to which each belongs. These colors shade and blend into thousands of combinations, but the following table will perhaps give you a fair idea of the subject, and will enable you more readily to understand what we will say a little later on in this lesson.

Auric Colors and Their Meanings.

Black represents hatred, malice, revenge, and similar feelings.

Gray, of a bright shade, represents selfishness.

Gray, of a peculiar shade (almost that of a corpse), represents fear and terror.

Gray, of a dark shade, represents depression and melancholy.

Green, of a dirty shade, represents jealousy. If much anger is mingled with the jealousy, it will appear as red flashes on the green background.

Green, of almost a slate-color shade, represents low deceit.

Green, of a peculiar bright shade, represents tolerance to the opinions and beliefs of others, easy adjustment to changing conditions, adaptability, tact, politeness, worldly wisdom, etc., and qualities which some might possibly consider "refined deceit."

Red, of a shade resembling the dull flame when it bursts out of a burning building, mingled with the smoke, represents sensuality and the animal passions.

Red, seen in the shape of bright-red flashes resembling the lightning flash in shape, indicates anger. These are usually shown on a black background in the case of anger arising from hatred or malice, but in cases of anger arising from jealousy they appear on a greenish background. Anger arising from indignation or defense of a supposed "right," lacks these backgrounds, and usually shows as red flashes independent of a background.

Crimson represents love, varying in shade according to the character of the passion. A gross sensual love will be a dull and heavy crimson, while one mixed with higher feelings will appear in lighter and more pleasing shades. A very high form of love shows a color almost approaching a beautiful rose color.

Brown, of a reddish tinge, represents avarice and greed.

Orange, of a bright shade, represents pride and ambition.

Yellow, in its various shades, represents intellectual power. If the intellect contents itself with things of a low order, the shade is a dark, dull yellow; and as the field of the intellect rises to higher levels, the color grows brighter and clearer, a beautiful golden yellow betokening great intellectual attainment, broad and brilliant reasoning, etc.

Blue, of a dark shade, represents religious thought, emotion, and feeling. This color, however, varies in clearness according to the degree of unselfishness manifest in the religious conception. The shades and degrees of clearness vary from a dull indigo to a beautiful rich violet, the latter representing the highest religious feeling.

Light Blue, of a peculiarly clear and luminous shade, represents spirituality. Some of the higher degrees of spirituality observed in ordinary mankind show themselves in this shade of blue filled with luminous bright points, sparkling and twinkling like stars on a clear winter night.

The student will remember that these colors form endless combinations and blendings, and show themselves in greatly varying degrees of brightness and size, all of which have meanings to the developed occultist.

In addition to the colors mentioned above, there are several others for which we have no names, as they are outside of the colors visible in the spectrum, and consequently science, not being able to perceive them, has not thought it necessary to bestow definite names upon them, although theoretically they are known to exist. Science tells us that there exist what are known as "ultra-violet" rays and "ultra-red" rays, neither of which can be followed by the human eyes, even with the aid of mechanical appliances, the vibrations being beyond our senses. These two "ultra" colors (and several others unknown to science) are known to occultists and may be seen by the person of a certain degree of psychic power. The significance of this statement may be more fully grasped when we state that when

seen in the Human Aura either of these "ultra" colors indicates psychic development, the degree of intensity depending upon the degree of development.
Another remarkable fact, to those who have not
thought of the matter, is that the "ultra-violet" color
in the Aura indicates psychic development when
used on a high and unselfish plane, while "the ultra-
red" color, when seen in the Human Aura, indicates
that the person has psychic development, but is using
the same for selfish and unworthy purposes—"black
magic," in fact. The "ultra-violet" rays lie just outside of an extreme of the visible spectrum known
to science, while the "ultra-red" rays lie just beyond
the other extreme. The vibrations of the first are
too high for the ordinary human eye to sense, while
the second consists of vibrations as much too low as
the first is too high. And the real difference between the two forms of psychic power is as great as
is indicated by the respective positions of these two
"ultra" colors. In addition to the two "ultra" colors
just alluded to, there is another which is invisible
to the ordinary sight — the *true* primary yellow,
which is indicative of the Spiritual Illumination
and which is faintly seen around the heads of the
spiritually great. The color which we are taught is
characteristic of the seventh principle, Spirit, is said
to be of pure white light, of a peculiar brilliancy,
the like of which has never been seen by human
eyes—in fact, the very existence of *absolute* "white

light" is denied by Western science.

The Aura emanating from the Instinctive **Mind** consists principally of the heavier and duller shades. In sleep, when the mind is quiet, there appears chiefly a certain dull red, which indicates that the Instinctive Mind is merely performing the animal functions of the body. This shade, of course, is always apparent, but during the waking hours is often obscured by the brighter shades of the passing thoughts, emotions, or feelings.

Right here it would be well to state that even when the mind is calm there hover in the Aura the shades indicative of the predominant tendencies of the man, so that his stage of advancement and development as well as his "tastes" and other features of his personality may be easily distinguished. When the mind is swept by a strong passion, feeling, or emotion, the entire Aura seems to be colored by the particular shade or shades representing it. For instance, a violent fit of anger causes the whole Aura to show bright red flashes upon a black background, almost eclipsing the other colors. This state lasts for a longer or shorter time, according to the strength of the passion. If people could but have a glimpse of the Human Aura when so colored, they would become so horrified at the dreadful sight that they would never again permit themselves to fly into a rage—it resembles the flames and smoke of the "pit" which is referred to in certain orthodox churches, and, in fact, the human mind in such a condition becomes a veritable hell temporarily. A strong wave of love sweeping over the mind will cause the entire Aura to show crimson, the shade depending upon the character of the passion. Likewise, a burst of religious feeling will bestow upon the entire Aura a blue tinge, as explained in the table of colors. In short, a strong emotion, feeling, or passion causes the entire Aura to take on its color while the feeling lasts. You will see from what we have said that there are two aspects to the color feature of the Aura; the first depending upon the predominant thoughts habitually manifesting in the mind of the person; the second depending upon the particular feeling, emotion, or passion (if any) being manifested at the particular time. The passing color disappears when the feeling dies away, although a feeling, passion, or emotion repeatedly manifested shows itself in time upon the habitual Auric color. The habitual color shown in the Aura, of course, changes gradually from time to time as the character of the person improves or changes. The habitual colors shown indicate the "general character" of the person; the passing colors show what feeling, emotion, or passion (if any) is dominating him at that particular time.

The student who has read the preceding lessons will realize readily that as the man develops and unfolds he becomes less and less the prey of passing passions, emotions, or feelings emanating from the

Instinctive Mind, and that Intellect, and then Spiritual Mind, manifest themselves instead of lying dormant in a latent condition. Remembering this, he will readily see how great a difference there must be between the Aura of an undeveloped man and that of the developed man. The one is a mass of dull, heavy, gross colors, the entire mass being frequently flooded by the color of some passing emotion, feeling, or passion. The other shows the higher colors and is very much clearer, being but little disturbed by feelings, emotion, and passions, all of which have been brought largely under the control of the will.

The man who has Intellect well developed shows an Aura flooded with the beautiful golden yellow betokening intellectuality. This color in such cases is particularly apparent in the upper part of the Aura, surrounding the head and shoulders of the man, the more animal colors sinking to the lower part of the Aura. Read the remarks under the head of "Yellow" in the color table in this lesson. When the man's Intellect has absorbed the idea of spirituality and devotes itself to the acquirement of spiritual power, development, and unfoldment, this yellow will show around its edges a light blue of a peculiarly clear and luminous shade. This peculiar light blue is indicative of what is generally called "spirituality," but which is simply "intellectual-spirituality," if you will pardon the use of the some-

what paradoxical term—it is not the same thing as
Spiritual Mind, but is merely Intellect impregnated
by Spiritual Mind, to use another poor term.   In
some cases of a high development of this intellectual
state, the luminous light blue shows as a broad fringe
or border often being larger than the center itself,
and in addition, in special cases, the light blue is
filled with brilliant luminous points, sparkling and
twinkling like stars on a clear winter night.   These
bright points indicate that the color of the Aura of
the Spiritual Mind is asserting itself, and shows that
Spiritual Consciousness has either been made mo-
mentarily evident to the man or is about to be made
so in the near future.   This is a point upon which
much confusion has arisen in the minds of students
and even teachers of occultism.   The next paragraph will also have some bearing upon the matter.

The Aura emanating from the Spiritual Mind, or
sixth principle, bears the color of the *true* primary
yellow, which is invisible to ordinary sight and
which cannot be reproduced artificially by man.   It
centers around the head of the spiritually illu-
mined, and at times produces a peculiar glow which
can even be seen by undeveloped people.   This is
particularly true when the spiritually developed
person is engaged in earnest discourse or teaching,
at which times his countenance seems fairly to
glow and to possess a luminosity of a peculiar kind.
The nimbus shown in pictures of the great spir-

itual leaders of the race is the result of a tradition arising from a fact actually experienced by the early followers of such leaders. The "halo" or "glory" shown on pictures arises from the same fact. When we again look upon Hoffman's wonderful picture, "Gethsemane," we will experience a new understanding of the mystic glow around the head of the great spiritual Teacher whose deep and true teachings have been obscured from the minds of many of those who claim His name, by reason of the ignorance of the generations of teachers who have lived since His death, but whose teachings are a living truth to occultists of all races. lands, and outward apparent differences of belief.

Of the Aura of the seventh principle, Spirit, we can say but little, and that little has been handed down to us by tradition. We are told that it consists of a "pure white" light, something unknown to science. No man among us has ever seen this light and none of us ever will (in this stage of development). The sight of this wonderful effulgence is reserved for beings far higher in the scale than are we, but who were once mortals like unto us, and like whom we shall in due time be. "We are Sons of God, and it doth not yet appear what we shall be"; but we are on The Path, and Those who have gone before send back cheering messages to us. After long ages we are going home.

THE FIFTH LESSON.

Thought Dynamics.

Had these lessons been written twenty years ago, instead of to-day, it would have been a most difficult task to have awakened the understanding of the Western public to the importance of the power of thought, its nature, its effects. Twenty years ago but comparatively few people in the Western world knew anything about the subject in question, and, outside of a few occultists, the words of the teacher would have been regarded as the wildest utterances. But, during the time mentioned, the Western world has been slowly educated to at least a partial understanding of the power of thought, and echoes of the great Oriental teachings on this subject have reached the ears of nearly every thinking person in the Western world, this being particularly true of Great Britain and America.

This awakening is in accordance with natural laws, and is a part of the evolution of the race. It is true that much of the teaching has come from persons who have had but a partial awakening to the truth, and consequently the teachings have been

73

more or less crude and imperfect and more or less colored by the personal theories and speculations of the various teachers who have been writing and speaking upon the subject. The average Western student, who has been interested in the various movements which may be roughly grouped together under the style of "The New Thought," has been more or less confused by the apparently conflicting theories and teachings which have resulted from the various speculations and theories of the numerous teachers who have sprung up, grown, and in many cases afterward "gone to seed." But a careful analysis will show that underlying all of the teachings are certain fundamental facts which the awakened mind grasps as truth. All of these teachers have done good work, and, in fact, the teachings of each have reached certain minds which needed the particular thing taught by the particular teacher, and which teaching was the very best possible, considering the particular stage of development of the student. Many students have obtained much good from certain teachers, and have then grown beyond the teacher and his teaching, and have in turn become teachers themselves, giving forth to others the truth as it came to them, more or less colored by their own personality.

The careful student who has taken the trouble to run down to fundamental principles the teachings of these new schools of thought, will have discovered that they all rest upon the Oriental teachings which reach back beyond written history, and which have been the common property of occultists of all ages and races. This "New Thought" is really the oldest thought, but the modern presentation of it comes as a new thing to those who hear it to-day, and the new movement is entitled to full credit for its work, and the advanced occultist knows that the fundamental truth lying underneath all of these conflicting theories will be gradually uncovered and brought to light, the speculations and pet theories of the various teachers being thrown aside.

The majority of those who read this lesson will have heard something of this subject of the power of thought, and will have doubtless had many experiences of its effect. So this lesson may come as an old story to nearly all of the members of the Class, but we will endeavor to give a brief, plain outline of the Yogi teachings upon the subject, which may help to reconcile some of the apparently conflicting theories which have been previously considered.

We shall not attempt to explain what thought *is* —that is too complicated a subject for elementary lessons. But we will begin by explaining some of its properties, laws, and effects. We avoid the theory for the time being, and get down to the "practical" side of the question.

You will remember what we said in our last lesson about the Aura. We explained that the Aura was projected into space by the several principles of man, just as is the light of the sun, the heat of a stove, the odor of a flower, etc. Each of these sources throws off vibrations, which we call light, heat, or odor, respectively. In one sense these emanations are minute particles of the thing which throws them off. In this connection we must also remember that the thing throwing off the emanations may be afterward withdrawn, but the emanations still remain for a greater or lesser time. For instance, astronomy teaches that a distant star may be destroyed, and yet the light rays thrown off from it will continue on their journey, and may soon be seen by us of the Earth years and years after the star itself has been destroyed—in fact, what we really see at any time are the rays of the star which left it many years before, the time, of course, depending upon the distance of the star from the earth. In the same way a fire in a stove may be extinguished, and yet the heat will remain in the room for a long time afterward. Likewise, a small particle of musk may be exposed in a room and then removed, and yet the odor will be perceptible for a long time. In the same way thoughts may be in active existence which have been sent out years before by some person, whose entire mental character may have changed or who, in fact, may have passed out of the body long since. Places and localities are often permeated by the thought of persons who formerly lived there, who have moved away or died many years ago.

The mind is continually throwing off emanations, which may be seen as the Aura extending a few feet from the person, and which usually becomes thinner and less easily perceived as it extends away from the sender. We are constantly sending forth thought-waves (to use a favorite term), and these waves, after the initial force of projection is expended, float along like clouds, mixing with other thought-waves of the same character, and extending often to far distant parts of the earth. Some of the thought emanations remain around the place from which they were sent forth, and unless disturbed by strong thoughts of a contrary nature will remain but slightly changed for many years. Other thoughts sent forth with a definite purpose or under a strong desire, emotion, or passion, will go forth rapidly toward the object to which they are directed. We shall see instances of this as we proceed with this lesson.

The majority of persons put very little force into their thought; in fact, thinking with them becomes almost a mechanical process, and consequently their thought-waves have very little motion imparted to them and do not travel very far, unless drawn by some other person of similar thought who attracts them to him. (We are merely stating general principles as we go along, repeating them when necessary, so that the student will gradually absorb the idea. We consider this conversational method the

most effective form of teaching—far more so than
the usual "cut-and-dried" form.)

We wish the student to particularly understand
that when we say "Thoughts are Things," we are
not using the words in a figurative sense or in a fan-
ciful way, but that we are expressing a literal truth.
We mean that thought is as much a "thing" as is
light, heat, electricity, or similar forms of manifestations. Thought can be seen by the psychic sight;
can be felt by the sensitive; and, if the proper instruments were in existence, could be weighed.
Thought, after being sent forth, is of a cloudy appearance, bearing the color belonging to it, as described in our lesson on the Aura. It is like a thin
vapor (the degree of density varying), and is just as
real as the air around us or the vapor of steam or
the numerous gases with which we are acquainted.
And it has power, just as have all of these forms of
vapor which we have just mentioned.

In this place let us mention that when a thought
is sent forth with strength, it usually carries with it
a certain amount of Prana, which gives it additional
power and strength, and often produces startling
effects. The Prana practically "vitalizes" it in some
cases, and makes of it almost a living force. We
will have more to say on this point a little later on.

So, friends and students, please remember always
that when we speak of thoughts being real things,
we mean just what we say. It may be necessary for

you to fix this fact in your minds by picturing the mind as sending forth thought emanations. Some find the picture of the throwing off of light-waves an easy way to fix the idea in their minds. Others prefer the illustration of the throwing off of heat by a stove. Others find it easier to think of a flower throwing off a strong perfume. And one student (now far advanced) preferred to think of thought emanations as akin to the steam being projected from a boiling tea-kettle. Take your choice or invent illustrations of your own, but get the idea fixed in your minds some way. It is much easier to work out these things by means of a material illustration than to attempt to carry an abstract idea in the mind.

While, as a rule, the power of thought of a certain kind depends upon the strength with which it has been projected, there is another element of strength which enables thoughts to manifest power. We allude to the tendency of thought to attract to itself other thoughts of a similar nature and thus combine force. Not only does thought along any lines tend to attract to the thinker corresponding thought attracted from the thought-atmosphere within the field of attraction, but thoughts have a tendency to flock together—to coalesce, to blend together. The average thought-atmosphere of a community is the composite thoughts of the people composing that community. Places, like persons, have their peculiarities, their characteristics, their strong and weak points, their prevailing atmosphere. This fact is apparent to all who have thought at all upon these lines, but the matter is usually dismissed without any attempt at explanation. But it must be apparent that the place itself is not an entity, and that these characteristics are not inherent in them, but must have some cause or origin. The occultist knows that this thought-atmosphere of a village, town, city, or nation is the composite thought of those dwelling in it or who have previously dwelt there. Strangers coming into the community feel the changed atmosphere about it, and, unless they find it in harmony with their own mental character, they feel uncomfortable and desire to leave the place. If one, not understanding the laws operating in the thought world, remains long in a place, he is most likely to be influenced by the prevailing thought-atmosphere, and in spite of himself a change begins to be manifest in him and he sinks or rises to the level of the prevailing thought.

In the older countries the characteristics of the leading cities of the nation have grown more or less alike, although there are still many points of difference which the stranger at once feels when he visits them. But in America, where the country is larger and newer, the differences to be noticed in localities are most marked. This is true not only in different sections of the country, but in cities near each other. Let the thoughtful stranger visit in turn the leading

cities of the United States, and he will be struck
with the spirit of each place, each having its own
personality and characteristics, the result of certain
lines of thought on the part of the early settlers of
the place, which in turn affected the new-comers,
who added their thought emanations to the atmosphere of the place, and so on, from time to time,
until the several cities have grown farther apart in
their characteristics than have many different na-
tionalities. Let the stranger visit in turn, say Boston,
New York, Philadelphia, Chicago, Denver, and San
Francisco, and he will notice the greatest differences
in the characteristics of each place. This difference
does not appear so strongly when he talks to individual citizens, but is quite noticeable when he
opens himself up to the "spirit of the place." People
often speak of these characteristics as "the air" of
the place, and the real explanation has been given
above—it is the thought-atmosphere of the town.
These characteristics may be modified or even
greatly changed by a new set of people settling in a
town. A few energetic thinkers will send forth
strong waves of thought in their every-day life, which
will soon color the composite thought of the place.
The thought of one strong thinker will overcome
the weak, purposeless thought of very many people
who send forth only negative thoughts. The positive is a sure antidote to the negative. In the same
way the "spirit" of the nation is a composite of the

"spirit" of its several parts. If one removes to a
town in which the greatest energy is being manifested, he soon feels the effect of the positive thought
around him, which awakens similar thoughts within himself. If one removes to a sleepy, "dead" community, his activities will become deadened and he
will gradually sink to the level of the town. Of
course, the man or woman who has built up a
strong, positive individuality will not be affected so
easily as the one of opposite characteristics, and, in
fact, he may even act as a leaven for the mass; but in
a general way the average person is greatly influenced by the composite thought-atmosphere of the
locality in which he spends most of his time.

In the same way dwellings, business-places, build-
ings, etc., take on the predominant thought of those
inhabiting them or who have dwelt in them. Some
places are notoriously "unlucky," and, although this
condition may be reversed by the man or woman of
strong will, the average person is affected by it.
Some houses carry with them an atmosphere of sun-
shine, good-fellowship, and good cheer, while others
are cold and repellent. A place of business is very
apt to reflect the prevailing thought of those at the
head of the enterprise or those who direct its affairs.
Certain shops inspire confidence in patrons, while
others cause one to keep a tight clutch on the
pocketbook and a close eye on the clerks.

Places in which crimes have been committed

often carry with them an unpleasant atmosphere, which originally arose from the strong thoughts sent forth from those participating in the occurrence, both the criminal and the victim. The atmosphere of a prison is horrifying to the sensitive. The atmosphere of a place of vice or scene of low animal pleasures is suffocating to one of higher mental traits. The atmosphere of a hospital is apt to influence those visiting it. The atmosphere of an old church is apt to produce in the mind of the visitor a feeling of quiet and calm. We are speaking in generalities, of course, as there are many influences modifying and changing these tendencies.

Thus it is with individuals. Some carry about them an atmosphere of cheer, sunniness, and courage, while others bring into a room a feeling of inharmony, distrust, and uneasiness. Many act as "kill-joys" and as dampers upon enthusiasm and free expression. Hundreds of instances illustrating this fact might be cited, but the student may supply these from his own experience and observation.

The various waves of thought sent forth by people attract and are attracted by thoughts of a similar character. They form thought strata in the astral space, just as clouds fall into groups in the atmosphere. This does not mean that each stratum of thought occupies a certain portion of space to the exclusion of all other thought clouds. On the contrary, these thought particles forming the clouds are of different degrees of vibration, and the same space may be filled with thought matter of a thousand kinds, passing freely about and interpenetrating, without interference with each other, but not assimilating except with thoughts of similar character, although temporary combinations may be formed in some cases. We cannot go into detail regarding this in this lesson, and merely wish to give the student a general idea of the subject, upon which he may build from time to time.

Each individual draws to himself the thoughts corresponding to those produced by his own mind, and he is of course in turn influenced by these attracted thoughts. It is a case of adding fuel to the fire. Let one harbor thoughts of malice or hate for any length of time, and he will be horrified at the vile flood of thoughts which come pouring into his mind. And the longer he persists in the mental state the worse matters will get with him. He is making himself a center for thoughts of that kind. And if he keeps it up until it becomes habitual to him, he will attract to himself circumstances and conditions which will give him an opportunity to manifest these thoughts in action. Not only does a mental state attract similar thoughts to it, but it leads the thinker into circumstances and conditions calculated to enable him to make use of these thoughts and inclinations which he has been harboring. Let one's mind dwell on the animal passions, and all nature will seem to conspire to lead him into position whereby these passions may be gratified.

On the other hand, let one cultivate the habit of thinking higher and better thoughts, and he will in time be drawn into conditions in harmony with the habit of thought, and will also draw to himself other thoughts which will readily coalesce with his own. Not only is this true, but each person will draw to himself other people of similar thoughts, and will in turn be drawn to them. We really make our own surroundings and company by our thoughts of yesterday or to-day. Yesterday's thoughts influence us to a greater or lesser extent, but to-day's thought will gradually supplant and drive out the cast-off thoughts of the past if we will that such shall be so.

We have said that thought charged with Prana manifested a much stronger force than the ordinary thought. In fact, all positive thought is sent forth charged with more or less Prana. The man of strong will sending forth a vigorous positive thought unconsciously (or consciously if he understands the subject) sends with it a supply of Prana proportioned to the force with which the thought was propelled. Such thoughts are often sent like a bullet to the mark, instead of drifting along slowly like an ordinary thought emanation. Some public speakers have acquired this art, and one can fairly feel the impact of the thought behind their utterances. A strong, vigorous thinker, whose thought is charged strongly with Prana, often creates what are known as Thought-Forms—that is to say, thoughts possessing such vitality that they become almost like living forces. Such thought-forms, when they come into one's psychic atmosphere, possess almost the same power that the person sending them would possess were he present, urging his thought upon you in an earnest conversation. Those high in occult development frequently send thought-forms to aid and help their fellow-beings when in distress or need, and many of us have experienced the effect of helpful thoughts sent in this manner while we did not dream of the cause of the changed feeling which came over us, bringing with it the consciousness of renewed strength and courage.

While thought-forms are aften sent out unconsciously by men of selfish desires and aims and many are affected by them, we wish to say that there need be no fear of any one being affected against his own good if he will maintain a mental atmosphere of Love and Confidence. These two conditions will repel the strongest thought-wave which may either be directed against one or which may be encountered in the astral atmosphere. The higher the order of thought the stronger it is, and the weakest person, providing his mind is filled with Universal Love and Confidence in the One Power, is many times stronger than the person of the strongest power who would stoop to use that power for selfish ends. The highest powers of this kind can be possessed only by those of great spiritual development, who have long since left behind them the low aims and ambitions of undeveloped man. Such persons are constantly sending forth thought-waves of strength and help, which may be drawn upon by those who need such help. All that one has to do is to make the mental demand for help from those who are able to give it, and at once they attract to themselves the waves of the strong, helpful spiritual thought which is being constantly emanated from the minds of the helpers of the race, both in the flesh and out of it. Were the race at the mercy of those of selfish thoughts, it would have perished long since, but things are otherwise ordered.

The only things to be feared in the world of thought-forms are those corresponding with any base thoughts which we may be entertaining ourselves. For instance, if we entertain low, selfish thoughts, we are open to thought-forms of similar character which may be lurking in the psychic atmosphere, which may take hold of our minds and urge us on to the doing of things which we would have shrunk from doing in the beginning. We have the right to invite what mental guests we wish—let us be careful to whom we issue invitations.

Our strong desires create thought-forms which

work toward the gratification of those desires, be they good or bad. We draw things toward us and are drawn toward things by these thought-forms. They become powerful helpers, and never sleep in their work. Let us be careful how we send them forth. Send forth no strong thought-desire unless it meet with the approval of the Highest Self. Otherwise you will become enmeshed in the consequences arising from it, and will suffer much in learning the lesson that psychic powers must not be used for unworthy ends. You are punished *by* such things, not *for* them. Above all, never under any circumstances send forth a strong desire-thought to injure another, for there is but one consequence of such an act and the experience will prove a bitter lesson. Such a person is usually hanged on the gallows he builds for others. Evil thought projected against a pure mind will rebound at once to the sender, and will gather force from the impact. We must apologize to our students for laying so much stress on these matters, but as there is always the chance of lessons of this kind falling into the hands of those unprepared to receive them, it is necessary for the warning to accompany anything written on the subject, in order to prevent thoughtless persons using the information improperly and thereby injuring themselves as well as others. It is the "Danger" signal displayed for the careless or thoughtless.

Those who have made a study of the dynamics of

thought are aware of the wonderful possibilities open for those who wish to take advantage of the stored-up thought which has emanated from the minds of thinkers in the past and present, and which is open to the demand and attraction of the one who may wish to use it and who knows how to avail himself of it.

There has been but little written on this phase of the subject, which fact is somewhat surprising when one considers the wonderful possibilities open to those who wish to take advantage of them. Much thought has been sent forth upon all subjects, and the man who is working along any line to-day may attract to himself most helpful thoughts relating to his favorite subject. In fact, some of the greatest inventions and most wonderful plans have come to some of the world's great people in this way, although those to whom they came have not realized from whence their information originated. Many a man has been thinking intently upon a certain subject, and has thrown himself open to the outside thought influences which have rushed toward his receptive mind, and lo! the desired plan—the missing link—came into the field of consciousness.

Unexpressed thought, originally sent out with considerable force of desire, constantly seeks for expression and outlet, and is easily drawn to the mind of one who will express it in action. That is to say, if an ingenious thinker evolves ideas which he has not the energy or ability to express in action, to take advantage of, the strong thoughts on the subject which he throws off will for years after seek other minds as a channel of expression; and when such thoughts are attracted by a man of sufficient energy to manifest them, they will pour into his mind like a flood until he seems to be inspired.

If one is working upon some problem which baffles him, he will do well to assume a receptive attitude toward thoughts along the same line, and it is extremely likely that when he has almost ceased to think of the matter at all the solution will flash before him as if by magic. Some of the world's greatest thinkers, writers, speakers, and inventors have experienced examples of this law of the thought world, although but few of them have realized the cause behind it. The astral world is full of excellent unexpressed thoughts waiting for the one who will express them and use them up. This is merely a hint of a great truth—let those make use of it who are ready for it.

In the same way one may draw to himself strong, helpful thoughts, which will aid him in overcoming fits of depression and discouragement. There is an immense amount of stored-up energy in the thought world, and any one who needs it may draw to himself that which he requires. It is simply a matter of demanding your own. The world's stored-up thought is yours—why do not you take it?

THE SIXTH LESSON.

TELEPATHY AND CLAIRVOYANCE.

Telepathy may be roughly defined as the communication of mind with mind, other than by means of the five senses to which material science limits man, viz: sight; hearing; smell; taste and touch—sight, hearing and touch being the senses most commonly used. According to material science, it would follow that if two minds were placed beyond the possibility of ordinary sense communication, there could be no communication. And, if there should prove to be communication under such circumstances, it would be a reasonable inference that man possessed senses other than the five which have been allotted him, or recognized in him, by material science.

Occultists, however, know that man has other senses and faculties than those taken into consideration by material science. Without going too deeply into this subject, and confining ourselves to the purposes of this lesson, we may say that besides the five physical senses he has five *astral* senses (counter parts of the physical senses), operating on the astral plane, by which he may see, hear, taste, and even feel, without the use of the physical organs usually associated with the use of these senses. More than this, he has a special sixth physical sense (for which we have no English term), by which he becomes aware of the *thoughts* emanating from the minds of others, even though the other minds may be far removed from him in space.

There is one great point of difference between this special sixth physical sense and the five astral senses. The difference is this: *The five astral senses are astral counterparts of the five physical senses, functioning upon the astral plane just as the five physical senses function upon the physical plane,* there being an astral sense corresponding with each physical organ, although the astral impression is not received through the physical organ, but reaches the consciousness along lines of its own, just as does the impression received through the physical channels. But this special sixth physical sense (let us call it "the telepathic sense," for want of a better name) *has both a physical organ through which it receives impressions,* and *also an astral sense counterpart, just as have the other physical senses.* In other words, it has an organ just as truly physical as is the nose, the eye, the ear, through which it receives the ordinary "telepathic" impressions, and which is used in all cases coming under the head of "telepathy." The astral counterpart is used on the astral plane in certain forms of clairvoyance. Now for the telepathic physical organ through which the brain receives the vibrations, or thought-waves, emanating from the minds of others.

Imbedded in the brain, near the middle of the skull, almost directly above the top of the spinal column, is to be found a small body, or gland, of reddish-gray color, cone-shaped, attached to the floor of the third ventricle of the brain, in front of the cerebellum. It is a mass of nervous matter, containing corpuscles resembling nerve cells, and also containing small concretions of gritty, calcareous particles, sometimes called "brain sand." This body is known to Western physical science as the "Pineal Gland," or "Pineal Body," the term "pineal" having been given it by reason of its shape, which resembles that of a pine-cone.

Western scientists are completely at sea regarding the function, purpose and use of this organ of the brain (for an organ it is). Their text-books dismiss the matter with the solemn statement, "the function of the pineal body is not understood," and no attempt is made to account for the presence and purposes of the "corpuscles resembling nerve cells," or the "brain sand." Some of the text-book writers, however, note the fact that this organ is larger in children than in adults, and more developed in adult females than in adult males—a most significant statement.

The Yogis have known for centuries that this

"Pineal Body" is the organ through which the brain receives impressions by the medium of vibrations caused by thoughts projected from other brains—the organ of "telepathic" communication, in short. It is not necessary for this organ to have an outward opening, as has the ear, nose and eye, for thought-vibrations penetrate matter of the consistency of the physical body, just as easily as light-vibrations penetrate glass, or X-ray-vibrations pass through wood, stone, etc. The nearest illustration of the character of thought-vibrations is found in the vibrations sent forth and received in "wireless telegraphy." The little "pineal body" of the brain is the receiving instrument of the wireless telegraphy of the mind.

When one "thinks" he sets up vibrations of greater or lesser intensity in the surrounding ether, which radiate from him in all directions, just as light-waves radiate from their source. These vibrations striking upon the telepathic organ in other brains cause a brain action which reproduces the thought in the brain of the recipient. This reproduced thought may pass into the field of consciousness, or it may remain in the region of the Instinctive Mind, according to circumstances.

In our last lesson, *"Thought Dynamics,"* we spoke of the influence and power of thought, and we suggest that, after finishing the present lesson, the student re-read the Fifth Lesson, in order to fix the two lessons together in his mind. In the previous lesson we told *what* thought-waves did—in this one we tell *how* they are received.

Telepathy then, for the purpose of this lesson, may be considered as the receiving by a person, consciously or unconsciously, of vibrations, or thought-waves, sent forth, consciously or unconsciously, from the minds of others. Thus, deliberate thought-transference between two or more people is Telepathy; and so, also, is the absorption by a person of the thought-vibrations in the atmosphere sent out by other thinkers without any desire to reach him. Thought-waves vary in intensity and force, as we have explained in the previous lesson. Concentration upon the part of the sender or receiver, or both, of course greatly intensifies the force of the sending, and the accuracy and clearness of the receiving.

CLAIRVOYANCE.

It is very difficult for us to speak intelligently of the phenomena coming under the head of Clairvoyance without getting into the subject of the Astral Plane, as Clairvoyance is an incident of the Astral Plane and belongs to that subject. But we cannot go into details regarding the Astral Plane, as we intend to devote an entire lesson to that subject, so we must go on with the subject before us, with the understanding that the student will be given an explanation of the nature and incidents of the Astral

Plane in due time. For the purpose of this lesson, however, we must ask the student to accept the statement that man has within him faculties which enable him to "sense" vibrations which are not responded to by his ordinary physical organs of sense. Each physical sense has its corresponding astral sense, which is open to the vibrations alluded to and which interpret such vibrations and pass them on to the consciousness of man.

Thus, the astral sight enables man to receive astral light-vibrations from an enormous distance; to receive these rays through solid objects; to perceive thought-forms in the ether, etc. Astral hearing enables one to receive astral sound-vibrations from enormous distances, and after a long time has elapsed, the fine vibrations still remaining in existence. The other astral senses correspond to the other physical senses, except that like the astral senses of seeing and hearing they are an *extension* of the physical senses. We think that the matter was well, if rather crudely, expressed to us several years ago, by an uneducated psychic, who, after endeavoring to explain the resemblance of her astral senses to her physical ones, at last said, awkwardly: "The astral senses are just the same as the physical ones—*only more so.*" We do not think that we can improve upon the explanation of this uneducated woman.

All persons have the astral senses alluded to, but comparatively few have developed them so that they can consciously use them. Some have occasional flashes of astral sensing, but are not conscious of the source of their impressions, they merely knowing that "something came into their mind," and often dismissing the impression as an idle fancy. Those awakening into astral sensing are often as clumsy and awkward as is the infant when the physical senses begin to receive and translate impressions. The infant has to gauge distance in receiving impressions through the eye and ear, and also in the matter of touch. The infant in psychism has to pass through a similar experience, hence the confusing and unsatisfactory results at the beginning.

SIMPLE CLAIRVOYANCE.

In order to intelligently understand the several forms of clairvoyant phenomena, more particularly those forms which manifest in what we will call "space clairvoyance," *i. e.*, the power to see things at great distances, we must accept as facts the occult teachings (which the latest discoveries of modern physical science are verifying) that all forms of matter are constantly throwing forth radiations in all directions. These astral rays are many times more subtle and fine than ordinary light rays, but they travel in the same manner and are caught up and registered by the astral sense of sight just as are ordinary light rays by the physical organs of sight. Like ordinary light rays these astral light rays move on infinitely, and the highly developed and trained astral senses of the advanced occultist register impressions from distances incredible to the average reader who has not studied these matters. These astral light rays penetrate and pass through solid material objects with comparatively no difficulty, and the densest bodies become almost transparent to the trained clairvoyant vision.

In all of the several forms of clairvoyance herein noted, there are of course various degrees of clairvoyant power on the part of the clairvoyant. Some manifest extraordinary power, others average, and the majority possess only occasional and more or less rudimentary power of sensing on the astral plane. This is the case with simple clairvoyance as well as with the higher forms, which we will presently describe. Accordingly, one may possess some of the characteristics of simple clairvoyance and lack the others.

By simple clairvoyance we mean the power to receive astral impressions from near by, the clairvoyant not possessing the power to see distant things or to sense things occurring in the past or present. To the person possessing a full degree of simple clairvoyance there occurs the phenomenon of receiving astral light waves through solid objects. He, literally, sees things "through a stone wall." Solid objects become semi-transparent, and he senses the vibrations passing through them just as the observer with the proper apparatus senses the X Rays which have passed through a solid object. He is able to observe things transpiring in an adjoining room, and behind closed doors. He may read the contents of sealed letters, by practice. He may see several yards into the earth beneath his feet, and observe the minerals which may be there. He may see through the body of a person near him, and may also observe the working of the internal organs, and distinguish the cause of physical ailments in many cases. He may see the aura of persons with whom he comes in contact, observing the auric colors and thus ascertaining the quality of thought emanating from their minds. He may, by clairaudient power, hear things which are being said beyond the range of ordinary hearing. He becomes sensitive to the thoughts of others, owing to the exercise of his astral telepathic powers, which are many times keener than his ordinary telepathic senses. He may see disembodied spirits and other astral forms, which will be explained in the lesson treating that subject. In short, a new world of impressions is opened out before him. In some rare cases persons possessing simple clairvoyance gradually develop the faculty of magnifying the size of small objects at will—that is, through their astral vision they are able to adjust the focus so as to bring the astral image of the object before them enlarged to any desired size, just as does the person using the microscope. This faculty, however, is quite rare, and is seldom found to have been developed spontaneously—the faculty usually being possessed only by those of advanced and developed occult powers. A variation of this faculty will be noticed under the head of space clairvoyance, which we take up next.

SPACE CLAIRVOYANCE.

There are several means whereby the psychic or developed occultist may perceive people, things, scenes and events far removed from the observer, and far beyond the range of the physical vision. Two of these means will come under the head of this lesson, the other methods belonging to the higher planes of life, and being beyond the power of any but the adepts and most advanced occultists. The two methods alluded to come, strictly speaking, under the head of space clairvoyance on the astral plane, and therefore form a part of this lesson. The first of these methods consists of what we have described as simple clairvoyance, on an increased scale, by reason of the development of the faculty of focusing upon far distant objects and bringing them to view by means of what occultists know as "the astral tube," which will be described in the following paragraphs. The second method consists in projecting the astral body, consciously or unconsciously, and practically observing the scene on the spot, through the astral vision. This method will also be described a little later on in this lesson.

We have described the astral light rays emanating from all objects by means of which the astral vision becomes possible. And under the head of simple clairvoyance we have told you how the clairvoyant may observe near-by objects through his astral vision, just as he may through his physical sight, the astral light rays being used in the one case, just as are the ordinary light rays in the other. But just as one is unable to perceive a far removed object through his ordinary physical vision, although the light rays are not interrupted, so is the simple clairvoyant unable to "see" far removed objects by means of his astral vision, although the astral light rays are uninterrupted. On the physical plane, man, in order to see things beyond his normal vision, must make use of the telescope. Likewise, on the astral plane, he must call into operation some assistance to the simple astral vision, in order to receive a clear impression of things far off. This assistance, however, comes from within his own astral organism, and consists of a peculiar astral faculty which acts as the lens of a telescope and magnifies the rays received from afar, rendering them sufficiently large to be distinguished by the mind. This power is "telescopic" in effect, although it is really by a variation of that "miscroscopic" faculty noted under the head of simple clairvoyance. This telescopic faculty varies very much in psychics, some being able to see but a few

miles, while others receive impressions just as easily
from all parts of the earth, and a few have been able
to occasionally perceive scenes on other planets.

This telescopic astral vision is usually operated in
connection with what occultists have called the
"astral telescope," which is akin to the "astral telegraph," "astral current," etc., all of which are but
variations of the "astral tube." The astral tube is
caused by the forming of a thought current on the
astral plane (held together by a strong supply of
prana projected along with the thought), which
current renders far easier the passage of astral vibrations of all kinds, whether they be telepathic thought-
vibrations, astral light-vibrations, or astral sound-
vibrations. It is the bringing of the observer and
the observed—the projector and the recipient—or
the two persons in harmony—into a closer condition
of *rapport*. The astral tube is the means whereby
quite a variety of psychic phenomena is made possible.

In the case of astral telescopic vision, or "space
clairvoyance," the clairvoyant, either consciously or
unconsciously, sets up an astral tube connecting him
with the distant scene. The astral light-vibrations
reach him more easily by this method, and the outside impressions are inhibited or shut out, so that
the mind receives only the impressions from the
point focused upon. These impressions reach the
clairvoyant, and are magnified by his "telescopic"
faculty and are then plainly perceived by his astral

vision. This "telescopic" faculty, remember, acts merely as the lens through which the astral light rays pass, and by which they are magnified to a size sufficiently large to be distinguished by the astral vision, just as the ordinary light rays are magnified for the ordinary vision by the lens of the telescope. The analogy is a very close one, and will help you to form a clear mental idea of the process.

The "astral tube" is usually formed by the will of the clairvoyant, or by his strong desire, which has almost as much force. At times, however, the conditions being favorable, any idle thought may cause the erection of the astral circuit and the clairvoyant will see scenes unthought of, or even unknown to him. The idle thought may have formed a connection with other psychic currents, or have been attracted in certain directions by any of a thousand and one psychic causes under the law of attraction and association; but the will of the operator is usually sufficient to shut out the careless adjustments and to establish a speedy connection with the desired person or place. Many persons have this faculty well under control; others find it coming and going spontaneously; others are devoid of it except under mesmeric influence, etc. Many have found the crystal ball, or similar object, an easy means of creating the astral tube, the crystal being used as a sort of starting point. Crystal-gazing is merely space clairvoyance by use of the astral tube, the scenes perceived by the observer being seen by this means. We have space merely to state the general principles of this great subject, in order to give the student an intelligent idea of the several forms of psychic phenomena. We regret that we have not the opportunity to relate the interesting instances of clairvoyant power which have been recorded by eminent writers on this subject, and which are well attested from a scientific point of view. However, we are not starting to prove the existence of clairvoyance to you—we must assume that you know it to be a fact, or at least not antagonistic to the idea. Our space must be devoted to a brief description and explanation of this phenomena, rather than to any attempt to prove its reality to sceptics. It is a matter which, after all, every man must prove to his own satisfaction by his own experience, and which no outside proof will establish.

The second method of seeing things far removed from us by space, consists in the projecting of the astral body, consciously or unconsciously, and practically observing the scene on the spot, by means of the astral vision. This is a more difficult and rarer method than the ordinary "astral tube" method, just described, although many persons travel in the astral and perceive scenes which they think are seen in a dream or "in the mind's eye."

We have described the astral body in a previous lesson. It is possible for one to project their astral body, or travel in their astral body, to any point within the limits of this planet, although very few people are conscious of their ability to so travel, and considerable practice and caution is necessary for the beginner. Once on the spot the astral traveler may see what is going on around him, and is not confined to the small scene to which the psychic using the "astral tube" is restricted. His astral body follows his desires or will, and goes where it is ordered. The trained occultist merely wishes to be at a certain place, and his astral travels there with the rapidity of light, or even more rapidly. Of course, the untrained occultist has no such degree of control over his astral body, and is more or less clumsy in his management of it. People often travel in their astral body in their sleep; a smaller number travel unconsciously in their waking moments, and a few have acquired the knowledge enabling them to travel consciously and at will in their waking moments. The astral body is always connected with the physical body by a thin, silklike, astral thread, and the communication between the two is maintained. We will have more to say on the subject of the astral body in our Tenth Lesson, which treats of the Astral Plane. We merely allude to it here, in order to explain that what is called clairvoyance is sometimes accomplished by its aid, although it is a higher form of psychic power than the other forms of clairvoyance mentioned by us so far.

Past Time Clairvoyance.

Time clairvoyance, so far as regards the sensing of past events, is not a rare faculty among advanced occultists—in fact, it may be termed a common one among such people. And the same faculty, imperfectly manifested, is found among many ordinary psychics who are not acquainted with the nature of their power. Among this last mentioned class of people time clairvoyance is more or less unsatisfactory because imperfect and misleading, from causes which will be seen presently.

The statement that one may see past events and scenes, even by astral vision, will readily be seen to require an entirely different explanation from that given of simple and space clairvoyance, for in the latter cases the clairvoyant sees that which is actually occurring somewhere at the time it is seen, or at least, a few seconds previous, whereas, in the latter case, the clairvoyant sees something which has occurred, perhaps ages ago, and after apparently all records of it have perished. Ah, that is just the explanation—"*apparently* perished." Occultists know that nothing ever perishes, and that there are in existence on the higher planes of matter, imperishable and unalterable records of every scene, act, thought, and thing that ever existed or occurred. These akasic records are not on the astral plane, but are on a plane far above it, but they are mirrored on the astral plane, just as the sky and clouds are reflected in the body of the lake, and the observer who cannot see the sky itself may see its counterpart in the water. And just as his vision may be distorted by the ripples and waves on the water, so may the astral vision of these records of the past become distorted and imperfect impressions by reason of the disturbances in the astral light. Occultists for ages have used "water" as a symbol of the astral light—do you see why?

These akasic records contain the "memory" of all that has passed, and he who has access to them may read the past as he may a book. But only the most advanced intelligences have free access to these records—or rather have the power to read them. But many have acquired a greater or lesser degree of power, which enables them to read more or less plainly from the reflections of these records in the astral plane. Those who have developed time clairvoyance are able to see these reflections of the records as scenes actually occurring before them, just as one hears from the phonograph the voices of people long since passed out of the body, and just as others may listen to our voices centuries hence. It is impossible to explain to beginners the nature of these records— we have no words to explain them— even we who write these words have but a partial understanding of the inner mystery of the akasic records—then how may we make ourselves plain to those who are still further back on the path than we are? We can think of but one illustration—and that an imperfect one. In the brain of every human being there are millions of cells, each containing the records of some past event or thought or action. We cannot find these records by the microscope, or by chemical test, and yet they are there, and may be used. The memory of every act, thought, and deed remains, during life, in the brain, although its owner may not always be able to call it up in recollection. Can you grasp the idea of the akasic record from this illustration? In the great memory of the Universe are registered and stored away the records of all that has gone before—those who have access to the records may read—and those who are able to see even the astral reflection of the records, may read with greater or less accuracy and skill. This is the best we can offer you in the way of explaining an unexplainable matter. Those who are ready for the truth hidden in these words will see a glimpse of it; others must wait until they are ready.

FUTURE TIME CLAIRVOYANCE.

Time clairvoyance, so far as "seership" or the seeing into the future is concerned, is even still more difficult to explain. We shall not attempt it, except to say that in the astral light there are to be found faint and imperfect reflections, the workings of the great law of cause and effect, or rather of the shadows cast before the coming events. Some few have the power of a closer viewpoint of the things causing these shadows or reflections, while more have a degree of psychic power enabling them to see with their astral vision these poor reflections, distorted and uncertain, by reason of the waves and ripples on the body of the lake of astral light. There are higher planes of power whereby a few in each age have been able to see partially into the future, but such powers are far above the poor astral plane faculties, which although quite wonderful to the untrained occultist, are not so highly viewed by those who have progressed well along the path. We almost regret to be compelled to pass over this part of the subject in so few words, and with a mere hint of even the small particle of the truth vouchsafed to even the advanced seeker of the way. But we know full well that all will receive the light needed by them, just the moment they are ready—not one moment later—not one moment sooner. All that can be done is for us to drop a word here—a hint there— a planting of the seed. May the harvest come soon and be a rich one.

CLAIRAUDIENCE.

Clairaudience is the hearing on the astral plane by means of the astral senses. Nearly all that we have said about Clairvoyance is equally true of Clairaudience, the only difference being that a different astral organ is used. Simple clairaudience is similar to past time clairvoyance; even future time clairvoyance has a shadow of a resemblance in clairaudient phenomena; the only difference between the two astral manifestations is that they are experienced through two different astral senses. Some

clairvoyants are also clairaudients, while others
lack the latter power. On the other hand, some
hear clairaudiently but are unable to see the astral
light. On the whole, clairaudience is a somewhat
rarer manifestation than is clairvoyance.

PSYCHOMETRY.

Just as we may sometimes recall an apparently
forgotten thing, by seeing something which is associated with that thing in our memory, so may we
sometimes be able to open up the astral reflection of
the akasic records of some particular scene or event
by touching some material associated with the event
or scene. There seems to be almost an affinity between a bit of matter and the particular portion of
the akasic records containing the past history of the
thing in question. A bit of metal, or stone, or cloth,
or hair will open up the psychic vision of the things
previously associated with it in the past. Or, on the
other hand, we may bring ourselves in rapport with
persons now living, by means of a particle of their
clothing, hair, or articles formerly carried by them,
the *rapport* condition thus established enabling us
to more easily set up the "astral tube." Psychometry
is merely one or more forms of clairvoyance, brought
into operation by means of some connecting link
between persons or things, or some object connected
with these persons or things. It is not a distinct
class of psychic phenomena, but is merely a variation of the other classes, sometimes combining several classes of clairvoyance in its manifestation.

How to Develop Psychic Powers.

We are often asked the question which is probably in the minds of the majority of our students, at least those who have not yet manifested any marked exhibition of psychic power: "How can one develop the psychic power which is latent within him?"

There are many methods of such development, a few of which are desirable; many of which are undesirable, and some of which are positively harmful.

Among the harmful methods are those in use among certain savage races, and which obtain even among misguided ones of our own race. We allude to such objectionable practices as the use of stupefying drugs, whirling dances, voodoo practices, repulsive rites of the black magicians, and other similar practices which we do not consider it wisdom to even mention. These practices aim to produce an abnormal condition similar to intoxication, and which, like intoxication and drug habits, only result in physical and psychical ruin. Those indulging in them do, it is true, develop a low order of psychic or astral power, but they invariably attract to themselves an undesirable class of astral entities and often open themselves up to the influence of a low order of intelligences, which wise men carefully avoid and refuse to entertain. We will do no more than to utter a warning against these practices and their results. Our work is intended to elevate our students, not to drag them down to the level of the black magicians.

Other practices, more or less undesirable, although

not absolutely harmful in the sense that we speak of the last mentioned ones, are more or less common among both the Hindus of a certain class and the Western peoples. We allude to methods of self-hypnotization and of hypnotization by others, in order to produce, or induce, a psychic condition in which the person is entitled to catch glimpses of the astral world. Gazing at some bright object until a trance-like condition is induced, or the repetition of some monotonous formula until a drowsy condition is produced, are among the methods of this class. In the same class we place the ordinary process of hypnotism by others for the same purpose. There is, of course, a higher form of "mesmerism" known to occultists, which is on an entirely different plane, but occultists are reluctant to use same, except in certain cases, where good may result, and such methods are not known to the ordinary operator, who, alas, too often is a person of imperfect occult knowledge and training and of a low degree of moral character. We caution our students against allowing themselves to be experimented with in this manner.

There are two methods of psychic development practiced by the Yogis, which we will mention here. The first and highest is the development of psychic powers by first developing the spiritual faculties and nature, when the psychic powers may be used with intelligence and power without any special training—the higher attainment carrying with it the lower. In other words, the Yogi, bent on spiritual attainment, contents himself with merely an intellectual acquaintance with psychic power, in passing on, and then after he has acquired the higher spiritual knowledge and development, he returns and uses the tools ready at his hand, the use of which he now understands. In the Fourteenth Lesson of this series we will point out the way of this development —the lesson will be entirely devoted to pointing out the way to spiritual attainment.

There is, however, another way whereby some students of the Yogi Philosophy develop psychic powers in themselves, preferring to gain this knowledge by experiment and experience before passing on to the spiritual plane. We have no fault to find with this course, providing the student does not regard psychic power as the end of attainment, and providing he always is inspired with worthy motives and does not allow the interest of the astral plane to divert him from the main object—spiritual development. Some of the Yogi students follow the plan of first mastering the body by the mind, and then mastering the Instinctive Mind by the Intellect under the direction of the will. The first steps in the mastery of the body have been spoken of by us in "Science of Breath," and will be more clearly brought out and added to in our forthcoming book, "Hatha Yoga." The mental control forms a subject in itself, and we trust to find time to write a little manual on the subject some time during the present year.

If the student wishes to experiment a little for himself, we suggest that he acquire self-control and practice Concentration, in the Silence. Many of you have already had exhibitions of psychic power, and you may practice along the lines corresponding to the manifestations you have already had. If it be Telepathy, practice with some of your friends and note results. A little practice will work wonders for you. If it be Clairvoyance, you may practice with a crystal, or glass of clear water, to assist in concentrating, and to form the beginning of the astral tube. If it be Psychometry, practice by picking up some object, such as a pebble, a coin, a key, etc., and sit quietly taking note of the fleeting impressions which at first will come but dimly before your mind. The description of the different classes of phenomena mentioned in this lesson will suggest methods and exercises for you.

But do not allow yourself to be carried away by psychic practices—they are interesting and instructive, but they are not essential things at this stage of development. Keep your mind fixed always on the goal—the end to be attained—the development of the Real Self—the realization of the I Am within you—and the still higher realization of your Oneness with All.

Peace be to thee, student. You have our loving thought and wishes for your welfare. If you ever feel the need of our sympathy and mental help, call for it in the great Silence, and we will respond.

THE SEVENTH LESSON.

HUMAN MAGNETISM.

Human Magnetism, as the term is used in these lessons, is a very different thing from that which the public generally terms "Personal Magnetism." Personal Magnetism is an attribute of the mind, and belongs to the subject of the Dynamics of Thought. Human Magnetism, on the contrary, is a manifestation of Prana, and belongs to that part of the general subject.

The term "Human Magnetism" is a poor one, but like many other such terms, is used for want of a better one, and to avoid the coining of new terms which would be likely to confuse the student. The Sanscrit contains terms perfectly fitting each phase of the subject, which terms have come into use as the knowledge of the subject grew. And such will be the case as the knowledge of this philosophy of the Orient becomes more generally known to the Western people—new terms, fitting to the subject, will spring into general usage, and the confusion which now exists will cease.

We prefer the term "Human Magnetism" to that

of "Animal Magnetism," as the latter is generally
confounded with some manifestations of Mesmerism. But this Human Magnetism is not the sole
property of Man, for the lower animals possess it
in a degree. There is this difference, however—
Man is able to consciously direct it by his will, and
through his Thought, while the lower animals use
it more or less unconsciously, and without intellectual aid, or under control of the Will. Both the
lower animals and man constantly throw off this
magnetism, or pranic energy, unconsciously, but
the developed or psychically educated man has the
force under his control, and can either repress it to
a great extent, or throw off greatly increased quan-
tities of it; and may also direct it to any special place
or spot. He can also use it in connection with his
thought waves, in order to give the same a greater
carrying power and strength.

At the risk of being charged with needless repetition, we wish to impress upon your minds that this
Pranic Energy, or Human Magnetism, is a very different thing from "thought-force" or any exhibition
of the power of thought, except that it may be used
in connection with thought-waves as above stated.
It is merely a blind force of nature, just as is electricity or similar forces, and may be used consciously or unconsciously; wisely or foolishly. It has
no intelligent action except as directed by the mind
of its user. "Human Electricity" would be a far

more appropriate name for it than is "Human Magnetism"—for it resembles Electricity far more than it does Magnetism.

With this explanation, we will continue the use of the term "Magnetism," asking that you always remember just what we mean by the term.

Human Magnetism is a form of Pranic Energy. We have said something about Prana in our First Lesson. Prana is the Universal Energy, and is found in varying forms, in all things, animate or inanimate. All forms of Force or Energy are but manifestations of Prana. Electricity is a form of Prana — so is the force of Gravitation — so is the Human Magnetism. It is one of the Seven Principles of Man, and is found in a greater or lesser degree in all human organisms.

Man extracts Prana from the air he breathes; the food he eats; the fluid he drinks. If he be deficient in Prana, he becomes weak and "lacks vitality," as the term goes. When his supply of Prana is sufficiently large for his needs, he becomes active, bright, energetic, and "full of life." We have given directions regarding the acquiring and storing up of Prana, by means of Breath, in our little book, "Science of Breath," and will give directions for its best absorption from the food and fluids, in our forthcoming book, "Hatha Yoga."

There is a great difference in the amount of Prana absorbed and stored up by different persons.

Some are surcharged with Prana, and radiate it like an electrical machine, causing all others with whom they come in contact to feel increased health, strength, life and vigor. Others are so deficient in Prana, that when they come into company of other persons, their depleted condition causes them to draw upon the Pranic supply of magnetism of the others, the result being that the other persons so drawn upon, are apt to feel uncomfortable and weak after the interview. Some people are practically vampires, and live upon the magnetism of others, unconsciously, usually, although some have acquired the knowledge that they may live on others' strength in this way, and practice their wicked arts consciously. This conscious use of their power is a form of black magic, and is attended with certain psychic penalties and punishments. But no one can be thus drawn upon, either by the unconscious demand of others, or by conscious design, after they have once learned something about this Human Magnetism, and its laws.

Human Magnetism, or Pranic Energy, is a most potent therapeutic force, and, in one form or another, it is found in the majority of cases of psychic healing. It is one of the oldest forms of natural healing, and it may be said to be almost instinctive in the race. A child who has hurt itself, or who feels a pain, at once runs to its mother who kisses the hurt part, or places her hand on the seat of the pain and in a few moments the child is better. When we approach one who is suffering, it is very natural for us to place our hands on his brow, or to pass our hand over him. This instinctive use of the hand is a form of conveying magnetism to the afflicted person, who is usually relieved by the act. The holding of a babe to its mother's bosom, is another instinctive act for the same purpose. The mother's magnetism goes out, propelled by her loving thought, and the child is soothed, rested, and strengthened. Human Magnetism may be thrown off from the system by means of a desire or thought, or it may be more directly passed to another by means of the hand; contact of the body; a kiss; the breath; and similar ways. We will speak of this matter, again, in our Eighth Lesson, on "Occult Therapeutics."

It is impossible to give a plain, clear explanation of just what this Human Magnetism is, unless we go into the deeper occult teachings, which are not fitted for the beginner. To tell what Human Magnetism is, we must explain what Prana is, and in order to tell what Prana is, we must go right to the root of the matter and discover the true nature and origin of "Force," something which modern physical science has failed to do, but which the deeper occult teachings are able to explain, at least to those who have reached that stage of understanding, by slow, laborious and gradual steps.

It may be urged that we are expecting too much when we ask students to accept as truth, the statement that there exists such a thing as Human Magnetism, or Pranic Energy, at all, when we cannot explain its real nature. Replying to this objection, we answer that there are many things which may be proven by their observed effects, although the thing itself cannot be explained in plain terms. Take Electricity, or Magnetism, for instance—we have their existence clearly proved to us every day, by their effects, and yet physical science tells us very little that can be understood, about their real nature. And so it is with this other exhibition of Pranic Energy—Human Magnetism—we must look to its effects for proof, rather than try to solve the mystery of the common source of all forms of force —Prana.

But, we have had it urged that whereas we can easily observe the effects and outward manifestation of Electricity and Magnetism, there are no such effects and manifestations of Human Magnetism, or Pranic Energy. This objection has always amused us, when we remember that every movement of the body, from the mighty effort of the giant, to the quiver of an eye-lash, is a direct effect and manifestation of this Human Magnetism or Pranic Energy.

Physical scientists call this thing "Nervous Force" or similar names, but it is the same thing that we have called Human Magnetism—a form of **Pranic Energy.** When we wish to raise a finger, we put forth an effort of the Will, if the desire be a conscious one—or an effort of the Instinctive Mind, if the desire be sub-conscious—and a supply of Human Magnetism is sent to the muscles controlling the movement of the finger. The muscles contract, and the finger raises. And so it is with every movement of the body, both on the conscious and sub-conscious plane of effort. Every step we take is caused by this same process—every word we utter is produced in this way—every tear we shed obeys the law —even the beating of the heart responds to the supply of Human Magnetism, propelled, in this last case, by the command of the Instinctive Mind.

The magnetism is sent over the nerves, just as is a telegraph message sent over the wires leading from the central office to all parts of the land. The nerves are its telegraph wires, and the current in the body always travels over these wires. And just as, until a very recent time, it has been thought impossible for messages to be sent without wires, so even to this day, do the physical scientists deny that this Human Magnetism (which they call Nervous Force) can be transmitted except over these wires of the nervous system. And just as the scientists have recently discovered that "wireless telegraphy" is a possibility, and a working truth—so have the occultists known for centuries that this Human Magnetism can be transmitted from person to person, through the astral atmosphere, without the need of the wires of the nerves.

Have we helped you to form a clearer idea of Human Magnetism?

As we have stated, Human Magnetism is taken up by the organism of man, from the air he breathes; the water he drinks; and the food he eats. It is extracted in Nature's laboratory, and stored up in his nervous system, in a chain of storage-batteries, of which the Solar Plexus is the central and chief store-house. From these storage-batteries, the magnetism is drawn by the mind and sent forth to be used for the thousands of purposes for which it is intended. When we say, "drawn by the mind," we do not mean that it must be necessarily drawn by an effort of the conscious mind, or will power,—in fact, not over five per cent of the amount used is so drawn, the remaining ninety-five per cent, being drawn and used by the Instinctive Mind, which controls the functions of the body—the workings of the internal organs—the processes of digestion, assimilation, and elimination—the circulation of the blood and the various functions of the physical body, all of which are wholly, or in part, under the control and care of the Instinctive Mind.

Nor must it be supposed that this magnetism is absent from any part of the body, at any time; or is absent until it is sent there by a distinct effort of the mind. The fact is that every part of the body contains a greater or lesser amount of magnetism at all times—the amount depending upon the general vitality of the person, which vitality is determined entirely by the total amount of Prana, or Human Magnetism in the system.

A brief consideration of the nervous system, with its nerve-cells, ganglia, plexi, etc., will be advisable, at this point, in order to gain a clearer idea of the processes of nature in its distribution of the supply of magnetism.

The Nervous System of man is divided into two great systems, viz., the Cerebro-Spinal System, and the Sympathetic System. The Cerebro-Spinal System consists of all that part of the Nervous System contained within the cranial cavity, and the spinal canal, viz., the brain and the spinal cord, together with the nerves which branch off from the latter. This system presides over the functions of animal life known as volition, sensation, etc. The Sympathetic System includes all that part of the Nervous System located principally in the thoracic, abdominal, and pelvic cavities, and which is distributed to the internal organs. It controls the involuntary processes, such as growth, nutrition, etc., under the supervision and direction of the Instinctive Mind.

The Cerebro-Spinal System attends to all the seeing, hearing, tasting, smelling, feeling, etc. It sets things in motion; it is used by the Ego to think

—to manifest consciousness and Intellect. It is the instrument by which the Ego is enabled to communicate with the outside world by means of the physical senses. This system has been likened to a great telephone system, with the brain as the central office, and the spinal column and nerves as cable and wires respectively.

The brain is a great mass of nerve tissue, and consists of three parts, viz., the Cerebrum, or brain proper, which occupies the upper, front, middle and back portion of the skull; the Cerebellum, or "little brain," which fills the lower and back portion of the skull; and the Medulla Oblongata, which is the broadened commencement of the spinal cord, lying before and in front of the Cerebellum.

The Cerebrum is the organ of the Intellect, and also of the unfolding Spiritual Mind—the organ of manifestation, remember, not the thing itself. The Cerebellum is the organ of the Instinctive Mind. The Medulla Oblongata is the upper enlarged part of the spinal cord, and from it and the Cerebrum branch forth the cranial nerves which reach to various parts of the head; to the organs of special sense, and to some of the thoracic and abdominal organs, and to the organs of respiration.

The Spinal Cord, or spinal marrow, fills the spinal canal in the vertebral column, or "backbone." It is a long mass of nerve tissue, branching off at the several vertebrae to nerves communicating to all parts of the body. The Spinal Cord is like a great telephone cable, and the emerging nerves are like the private wires connecting therewith.

The Sympathetic System is composed of a double chain of ganglia on each side of the spinal column, and scattered ganglia in the head, neck, chest, and abdomen. (A ganglion is a mass of nervous matter, including nerve cells.) These ganglia are connected with each other by filaments, and are also connected with the Cerebro-Spinal System by motor and sensory nerves. From these ganglia numerous fibres branch out to the organs of the body, blood vessels, etc. At various points, the nerves meet together and form what are known as plexi, or plexuses. The Sympathetic System practically controls the involuntary processes, such as the circulation, respiration and digestion.

Over this wonderful sytsem operates the Human Magnetism or Pranic Energy (or "Nervous Force," if you prefer the term of the physical scientists.) By means of the impulses from the mind, through the brain, the magnetism is drawn from its storage batteries, and sent to all parts of the body, or to any particular part of the body, over the wires of the nervous system. Without this magnetism, the heart cannot beat; the blood cannot circulate; the lungs cannot breathe; the various organs cannot function; in fact, the entire machinery of the body comes to a stop if the supply of magnetism be shut off. Nay, more, even the brain itself cannot perform its functions as the physical organ of the mind, unless a supply of Prana or magnetism be present. And yet, the physical scientists smile at the mention of the subject of "Human Magnetism," and dismiss it by giving it another name, "Nervous Force," but limiting its scope.

The Yogi teachings go further than does Western Physical science regarding one particular part of the nervous system. We allude to that which physical scientists call "the Solar Plexus," or "Abdominal Brain," and which they consider as merely one of a series of certain matted nets of sympathetic nerves which, with their ganglia are found in various parts of the body. Yogi science teaches that this Solar Plexus is really a most important part of the nervous system, and that it is the great storehouse of Prana, which supplies the minor storage-batteries, and the entire system. The Solar Plexus is situated in the Epigastric region, just back of the pit of the stomach, on either side of the spinal column. It is composed of white and gray brain matter, similar to that composing the other brains of man. It plays a much more important part in the life of man than is generally supposed. Men have been killed instantly by a severe blow over this region, and prize fighters recognize its vulnerability, and frequently paralyze their opponents by a blow over it. The name "Solar" is well bestowed, as, in fact, it does radiate energy and strength to all parts of the body, even the upper brains depending upon it for energy with which to work.

Just as the blood penetrates all parts of the system, by means of the arteries, and smaller blood vessels, terminating in tiny, fine hair-like vessels called capillaries, and the system is thereby kept supplied with rich, red blood, building up and repairing the cells of the body, and supplying the material required for that endless work of repair and rebuilding which is constantly going on in every part of the body, under the direction of that faithful servant, the Instinctive Mind—so does this Human Magnetism, or Pranic Energy, penetrate every portion of the system, by means of this wonderful and complex machinery called the Nervous System, with its complicated systems within systems of cables, wires, relays, storage-batteries, and the like. Without this magnetism there could be no life, as even the machinery and apparatus for the carrying on of the work of the circulation of the blood depends for motive power upon this Pranic Energy.

The healthy human body is filled from head to toe with this wonderful force, which keeps its machinery moving, and which is used not only on the physical but on the astral plane, as we shall see later on.

But, it must be remembered that the Instinctive

Mind is back of all this distribution, for it keeps up a continual demand and draught upon the storage batteries of the system for a sufficient supply of magnetism to supply all parts of the body, and only calls for a special amount in response to a sudden and immediate demand. But the Instinctive Mind regards the supply and demand question in this continuous draught upon the storage batteries, and the consequent sending forth of the magnetism to all parts of the body. It sends forth only a certain reasonable percentage of the amount stored up, otherwise it would soon bankrupt the system. If one has an abundant supply of magnetism, the Instinctive Mind is quite liberal in disbursing that amount, for it is no miser—it is merely prudent—and such a person fairly radiates magnetism, so that others coming in contact with him feel the healthy outpouring which leaps beyond the confines of the nervous system, and fills the astral atmosphere around him. We have described the human Aura in our Fourth Lesson, and in the same lesson have touched upon the Aura of the third principle, or Prana, which is practically the Aura of Human Magnetism.

This Aura may be felt by many, and seen by those having a certain degree of clairvoyant vision. In fact, a good clairvoyant may see the magnetism as it moves along within the nervous system of a person. When in or very near the body, it has a faint rosy tint, which leaves it as it moves away from the body. At a little distance from the body, it resembles a vapory cloud of the color and appearance of an electric spark, or rather of the radiations from an X-ray tube. Clairvoyants see spark-like particles of it being shaken from the finger-tips of those giving "magnetic treatments" or mesmeric passes. It is also seen by some persons who do not consider themselves clairvoyants, to whom it appears like the heated air arising from a stove, or from the heated ground; that is, like a colorless, vapory something, pulsating and vibrating.

A person of strong concentration or trained powers of thought, also throws off a considerable amount of magnetism along with the thought-waves emanating from his brain. In fact, all thought-waves are more or less charged with magnetism, but those of poor concentration and negative character throw off so little that we do not generally take it into consideration as compared to the heavily charged thought waves of the positive or developed person.

The great point of difference between the physical scientist and the occultist, is in the question of the possible transference of magnetism, or nervous force as the physical scientist calls it. The physical scientist insists that although the nervous force undoubtedly exists and does all within the body that the occultist claims, yet it is confined to the nervous systems, and cannot traverse their limits. He consequently denies the existence of much of the phenomena incident to Human Magnetism, and considers the occult teachings as fit only for visionary and imaginative people. The occultist, on the other hand, knows by experience that this magnetism, or nervous force, can and repeatedly does traverse the boundaries of the nervous system, and is projected, at times, to distances far remote from the person in whose system it was stored up. The proof of this occult teaching is to be found by anyone who will experiment for himself, providing he will divest his mind of prejudice and will be willing to accept facts as they are presented to him.

Before proceeding further, we wish to again remind our students that this Human Magnetism is merely a manifestation or form of Prana, and that Prana is not made to order by people to supply their needs. When one increases the amount of magnetism in his system, he does it not by making a fresh supply of it, but by drawing to himself an increased supply of Prana from the great source of supply, by breathing, eating, or drinking. The amount so absorbed or extracted from air, food, and fluid may be greatly increased by the mental desire, or will power as we will presently see. There is a certain amount of Prana in existence— this amount cannot be added to or diminished. It is unchangeable. It is Force.

In our Fifth Lesson, we told you that when a thought is sent forth with strength, it usually carries with it a considerable amount of Prana, or magnetism, which gives to it additional strength, and sometimes produces startling effects. This Prana, or magnetism, practically vitalizes the thought, and makes it almost a living force. All positive thought, good or bad, is more or less heavily charged with Prana or magnetism. The man of strong will sending forth a vigorous, positive thought unconsciously (or consciously, if he understand the subject) sends with it a supply of Prana, or magnetism, proportioned to the force or energy with which the thought is propelled. A thought sent forth when one is laboring under a strong emotion is likewise heavily charged with magnetism. Thoughts, so charged, are often sent like a bullet to the mark, instead of drifting along slowly like an ordinary thought emanation. Some public speakers have acquired this art, and send forth their words with such force that one can fairly feel the impact of the thought. A strong, vigorous thinker, whose thoughts are heavily charged with Prana, will sometimes impart such vitality to his thoughts that they will live for a time as Thought Forms—that is to say, will possess such vitality, from the Prana with which they are charged, that they will become almost like living forces. We may have something to say on this subject in our Lesson on the Astral World (Lesson X). Such Thought Forms, coming into one's psychic atmosphere, possess almost the same degree of power that would be experienced were the person present in person talking to you. Read over pages 85-88, Fifth Lesson, now that you have learned some little more about Prana, and you will get a clearer idea of Thought Forms.

Prana depends very considerably upon the desires

and expectations of the person, both in the matter of his absorption and its projection with a thought-wave. That is to say, that while every person absorbs more or less Prana every moment of his life, and this amount may be largely increased by following the Yogi teaching regarding breathing, eating and drinking, still the thought, or desire, or expectation of the person will greatly increase the amount of Prana absorbed. And, in like manner, will the desire or will of the person greatly multiply the force with which a thought is projected, as it largely increases the amount of Prana with which the thought is charged.

To speak more plainly: If one will form a mental image of the absorption of Prana, while breathing, eating or drinking, he will bring into operation certain occult laws which will tend to release a greater amount of Prana from its confining matter, and he will be greatly strengthened in consequence. Try the experiment of taking a few deep breaths, holding the mental image that you are absorbing a large amount of Prana with each inward breath, and you will feel an influx of new strength. This is worth trying when you feel tired and exhausted. Likewise, drink slowly a cupful of water, forming the mental image that you are extracting from the water a great supply of Prana which is stored up in it, and you will experience a similar result. Likewise, in eating, if you will masticate your food slowly, holding the mental image that you are extracting the strength of the Prana in the food, you

will receive a much greater per cent of nouris
and strength from the food than you would ı
ordinary way. These things are all helpfu
hope that you will try them, and use them w ..cn
you need them. Do not let the simplicity of these
things cause you to undervalue them.

The same law causes a thought projected with
the mental image that it is heavily charged with
Prana, to attain a greater velocity and force than
would an ordinary thought, and its potency will be
greatly increased by this practice. But be careful
not to send forth evil thoughts in this way. Read
your lesson on "Thought Dynamics" (Fifth Lesson) carefully, and heed the warnings contained
therein.

A number of interesting experiments along the
lines of Human Magnetism may be tried. If you
have a number of friends interested in this subject
you may try this experiment: Let a party sit around
in a circle, holding hands, and all concentrate their
minds on the common purpose of sending a Pranic
current, or current of magnetism, around the circle.
There must be a common understanding of the
direction, else some will be sending in one direction
and some in another, and the benefit of co-opera-
tion will be lost. A good plan is to send the current
in the direction of the movement of the hands of a
watch around its face, that is, pick out some person
to represent the figure XII, and then start the current moving in the direction of "right" from that
person. If the party is harmonious, and the condi-

tions are favorable, they will soon feel a faint tingling like a weak current of electricity moving through them. This practice, if moderately indulged in, will prove invigorating to all concerned in it, but we would not advise that the sittings be continued too long, as it might produce a sufficiently strong current that might be conducive to the production of psychic phenomena, which should not be too freely indulged in by those who are not familiar with the laws of psychic phenomena. We do not approve of indiscriminate, and unintelligent production of phenomena of this sort. One should learn something of the laws, before he attempts to produce phenomena.

Our little book, "Science of Breath," gives in condensed form, a number of methods of using Pranic force, or Human Magnetism, and we refer the student to that book, after he has finished this lesson. All of our publications dove-tail one into the other, and as each one is read others become plainer. Of necessity, we must condense our information, and must trust to a careful reading of all the lessons on the part of our students, in order that they may obtain the best results.

In order not to go over the same ground twice we must refer the student to "Science of Breath" for directions and exercises calculated to increase the absorption of Prana, and also for directions regarding its distribution.

Chapter XIV, of "Science of Breath," gives you some valuable information along these lines. In this chapter, Paragraph 2 furnishes a fine exercise for the increased absorption of Prana, and its distribution to all parts of the body, strengthening and invigorating all the cells, organs and parts of the body. This exercise will seem doubly valuable to you now that we have gone a little deeper into the subject of Prana or magnetism. Paragraph 3, of the same chapter, instructs you how to inhibit pain by the direction of Prana. Paragraph 4 instructs you in the directing of the circulation. Paragraph 5 gives you information on Self Healing, and Paragraph 6 gives you a short course on Healing of Others, which if followed carefully by you will make you a good "magnetic healer." Paragraph 7 instructs you in Distant Healing.

The next chapter, Chapter XV, gives you information regarding thought projection by means of sending distant thoughts charged with Prana; directions for forming a Protective Aura, which will enable you to resist the thoughts and Prana of others, if desired—this information is especially valuable, and we urge upon the student that he acquire this practice of forming a Protective Aura, as he will find it of use to him many times. Our Fifth Lesson also contains directions for the same thing, going a little more into detail than does "Science of Breath." Chapter XV of "Science of Breath" also tells you how to Re-charge yourself, and how to Re-charge others, with Prana; also how to charge water, and quite a number of valuable exercises and directions for the use of Pranic force, or Human Magnetism; much of which has, so far as we know, never been printed before.

A casual reader of these concluding lines might very naturally suppose that we were trying to sell "Science of Breath" to our students, by reason of these constant references to it. We beg to inform such casual reader of a fact, which all our students realize, without being told, and that is, that nearly every student of this Class has read "Science of Breath," generally before he has purchased this Course. Consequently, he is not a good subject for another sale of the same book, so we must be relieved of the suspicion of an inordinate desire to sell our books by means of praising them in our lessons. Our real reason for this repeated allusion to "Science of Breath" is that we have noticed that the average student, even though he had re-read the little book several times, does not begin to realize the large amount of information contained within its pages, until his attention is called to it. Then, we know that if he takes up the book, after our calling his attention to it, he will be able to understand this particular lesson much better by reason of the reference to the book. Likewise, he will understand the book better by reason of his having just read the lesson. We wish to keep hammering away at these ideas, until our students have firmly grasped them. These lessons are intended as lessons, not as mere interesting reading. They are intended to teach something—not merely to amuse our students.

So, if the student wishes to practice the workings of Pranic Energy or Human Magnetism, we cheerfully direct him to "Science of Breath," in which he will find enough to keep him busy for a while.

In our Lesson VIII, on "Occult Therapeutics," we will also give him some work to do, if he desires, with a few exercises new to him.

As we have before said, these lessons must be read and re-read, in connection with one another, as one lesson will throw light on another, and vice versa. They are all parts of the one thing—all stones going to build up the temple—each has its place, and each fits into the other.

To those among our students, who have not reached that state of perfect health which the Yogi Philosophy teaches is desirable, as it fits the body for use as a perfect instrument of the Ego—to those who are suffering from disease and ill-health—we urge the practice of increasing the supply of Prana, by means of the breath, the food, and the fluids, as stated in this lesson, and in "Science of Breath." A careful and constant practice of this absorption and storage of Prana will benefit every person, particularly those who are not in perfect health. Do not despise the body, as it is the Temple of the Living Spirit. Tend it well, and make a worthy instrument of it.

THE EIGHTH LESSON.

OCCULT THERAPEUTICS.

The student of the history of Man will find in the legends, folk-lore, and history of all peoples evidences of the fact that healing by some form of Occult practice has been followed by all races—all peoples—at all times. These various forms of occult therapeutics have varied from the revolting practices accompanying the grossest form of barbaric superstition, to the most refined form of procedure accompanying some of the fashionable metaphysical cults of to-day. These various forms of occult healing of disease have been attached to all forms of religion, from the degraded voodooism of Africa, to the highest forms of religion known to the world. All sorts of theories have been advanced to account for the cures which have resulted from all these forms of healing—all manner of creeds built around the fact that cures have been made. Priests, teachers and healers have claimed Divine powers, and insisted that they were the representatives of the particular deity which was worshipped in their respective countries, simply because they were able to perform cures of bodily ills. And, in nearly every case, these priests and healers have claimed the

cures as proof positive of the truth of the respective
religion or school of religious thought which they
favored; and at the same time insisted that all other
forms of religions or occult healing were bogus and
counterfeit, and that they, the said priests making
the claim, had the only "real thing"; dire penalties
being often threatened to those who dared to pat-
ronize any of the opposition healers or priests.

Human nature is much the same all over the
world, and in all times. We find the same rivalry
and claim of "the only real thing" existing to-day,
both in the case of the rival Voodoo doctors of
Africa and the polished leaders of the fashionable
metaphysical cults of America—and among all who
come in between these two poles. Alas for these
claimers of a monopoly of one of Nature's great
forces—these people who make cures in spite of their
theories, rather than because of them! Nature's
great recuperative force is as free as air and sun-
shine, and may be used by anyone who cares to do
so. It is not owned or controlled by any person,
cult or school—and no particular form of religious
belief is necessary to one in order that he may obtain benefit from it—God's children amuse themselves with many forms, sects, and creeds, but He
knows them all as his children and smiles at their
childish desires to form themselves into cliques of
"chosen people," attempting to shut out their
brethren from the common heritage.

It must have become evident to the student that
there must be some great principle underlying all

these varying forms of occult healing, because they *all* make cures in spite of the fact that each claims to have the only correct theory and denounces the theories of the others. There must be some great force which they are all using, blindly in many cases, and their differing theories and creeds which they have built up around their cures must be merely regarded as incidents of the use of the great healing force, and in no way the real explanation of the phenomena of occult healing. Any explanation to be worth a moment's attention must explain, or attempt to explain, *all* the various forms of occult healing—for all the various cults and schools make cures, and have done so in all ages—in spite of their creeds and theories.

The Yogi philosophers have for centuries past known and practiced various forms of occult therapeutics, and have studied deeply and thoroughly into the principles underlying the cures. But they have never deceived themselves into imagining that they had any monopoly of the matter—in fact their researches and experiments have convinced them that *all* healers are using a great natural force—the same in all cases, although applied and called into operation in various ways—and that the metaphysical theories, religious beliefs, claims of divine favoritism, etc., that have been built around this occult healing, have no more to do with it than they would have to do with electricity or magnetism, had they been built around these great forces instead of around the great healing force.

The Yogis realize that all forms of healing are but different means of calling into operation this great force of Nature—some forms being fitted for one case, and some for others—combinations being often used to suit some particular case.

The Yogis realize that Prana is the direct force used in all of these cures, although the Prana is called into operation in several different ways, as we shall see as we proceed. They teach that all forms of occult healing can be explained in this way—in fact they perform cures in nearly all the ways used by the great schools of occult therapeutics—and have for centuries—believing that the one theory underlies them all.

They divide the forms of healing into three general classes, viz:

(I) Pranic Healing, including what is known to the Western world as "magnetic healing," etc.; (II) Mental Healing, including the several forms of mental and psychic healing, including "absent treatments," as well as cures made under what is known as "the law of suggestion", etc.; (III) Spiritual Healing, which is a very rare form of healing, and is possessed by those of advanced spiritual attainment, and is a very different thing from that which is called by the same name by some of the "healers" of to-day. But under even the last advanced form of healing lies the same force, "Prana." Prana is the instrument by which the cure is effected, no matter what method is used, or who uses it.

In considering the subject of Occult Therapeutics, we must go back to the beginning. Before considering the question of cure we must look at the healthy body.

The Yogi Philosophy teaches that God gives to each individual a physical machine adapted to his needs, and also supplies him with the means of keeping it in order, and of repairing it if his negligence allows it to become inefficient. The Yogis recognize the human body as the handiwork of a great Intelligence. They regard its organism as a working machine, the conception and operation of which indicates the greatest wisdom and care. They know that the body IS because of a great Intelligence, and they know that the same Intelligence is still operating through the physical body, and that as the individual falls in with the working of the Divine Law, so will he continue in health and strength. They also know that when Man runs contrary to that law, inharmony and disease result. They believe that it is ridiculous to suppose that this great Intelligence caused the beautiful human body to exist, and then ran away and left it to its fate, for they know that the Intelligence still presides over each and every function of the body, and may be safely trusted and not feared.

That Intelligence, the manifestation of which we call "Nature" or "The Life Principle", and similar names, is constantly on the alert to repair damage, heal wounds, knit together broken bones; to throw off harmful materials which have accumulated in the system; and in thousands of ways to keep the machine in good running order. Much that we call disease is really a beneficent action of Nature designed to get rid of poisonous substances which we have allowed to enter and remain in our system.

Let us see just what this body means. Let us suppose a soul seeking a tenement in which to work out this phase of its existence. Occultists know that in order to manifest in certain ways, the soul has need of a fleshly habitation. Let us see what the soul requires in the way of a body, and then let us see whether Nature has given it what it needs.

In the first place, the soul needs a highly organized physical instrument of thought, and a central station from which it may direct the workings of the body. Nature provides that wonderful instrument, the human brain, the possibilities of which we, at this time, but faintly recognize. The portion of the brain which Man uses in this stage of his development is but a tiny part of the entire brain-area. The unused portion is awaiting the evolution of the race.

Secondly, the soul needs organs designed to receive and record the various forms of impressions from without. Nature steps in and provides the eye, the ear, the nose, the organs of taste and the nerves whereby we feel. Nature is keeping other senses in reserve, until the need of them is felt by the race.

Then, means of communication between the brain and the different parts of the body are needed. Nature has "wired" the body with nerves in a wonderful manner. The brain telegraphs over these wires instructions to all parts of the body, sending its orders to cell and organ, and insisting upon immediate obedience. The brain receives telegrams from all parts of the body, warning it of danger; calling for help; making complaints, etc.

Then the body must have means of moving around in the world. It has outgrown the plantlike inherited tendencies, and wants to "move on." Besides this it wants to reach out after things and turn them to its own use. Nature has provided limbs, and muscles, and tendons, with which to work the limbs.

Then the body needs a frame work to keep it in shape, to protect it from shock; to give it strength and firmness; to prop it up, as it were. Nature gives it the bony frame known as the skeleton, a marvelous piece of machinery, which is well worthy of your study.

The soul needs a physical means of communication with other embodied souls. Nature supplies the means of communication in the organs of speech and hearing.

The body needs a system of carrying repair materials to all of its system, to build up; replenish: repair; and strengthen all the several parts. It also needs a similar system whereby the waste, refuse matter may be carried to the crematory, burned up and sent out of the system. Nature gives us the life-carrying blood—the arteries and veins through which it flows to and fro performing its work—the lungs to oxygenize the blood and to burn up the waste matter. (See "Science of Breath." Chapter III.)

The body needs material from the outside, with which to build up and repair its parts. Nature provides means of eating the food; of digesting it; of extracting the nutritious elements; of converting it into shape for absorption by the system; of excreting the waste portions.

And, finally, the body is provided with means of reproducing its kind, and providing other souls with fleshly tenements.

It is well worth the time of anyone to study something of the wonderful mechanism and workings of the human body. One gets from this study a most convincing realization of the reality of that great Intelligence in nature—he sees the great Life Principle in operation—he sees that it is not blind chance, or haphazard happening, but that it is the work of a mighty INTELLIGENCE.

Then he learns to trust that Intelligence, and to know that that which brought him into physical being will carry him through life—that the power which took charge of him *then,* has charge of him *now,* and will have charge of him *always.*

As we open ourselves to the inflow of the great Life Principle, so will we be benefitted. If we fear it, or trust it not, we shut the door upon it and must necessarily suffer.

The student may well ask what has all this to do with Occult Therapeutics, and may complain that we are giving him a lesson in Hatha Yoga, in which latter statement he would be near the truth. But we cannot get away from the idea that there is that in Nature which tends towards keeping a man in perfect health, and we cannot help feeling that the true teaching is rather to instruct people how to keep well in the first place rather than to point out how they may get well after they have violated Nature's laws. The Yogis think that it is illogical to build up a cult around methods of healing—they feel that *if* cults must be built up let them rally around the centre of Health, allowing the curing of disease to be merely incidental.

In "Hatha Yoga", our forthcoming book, we will give the principles of the Yogi Philosophy of perfect health, in which is taught the doctrine that Health is the normal condition of man, and that disease is largely a matter of ignorance and the disobeying of natural laws of living and thinking. We will teach there that the healing power exists in every man, and may be called into operation consciously or unconsciously. Occult healing is merely the calling into play of this inner force within the individual (sometimes with the assistance of other individuals), and the opening up of the system to the recuperative energies already within itself.

All healing is occasioned by what we have called the "Vital Force" in the individual. The active principle of this Vital Force is, as we have explained, that manifestation of universal force—Prana. In order to avoid repetition we would refer you to "Science of Breath" and to "Lesson Seventh" of this course, for an explanation of the Nervous System and how Prana operates over it. Read over what we have said on this subject, and you will be able to more clearly understand what we are about to say regarding the different forms of occult healing.

Let us suppose that a person has neglected the rules of right living and thinking, as set forth in "Hatha Yoga" and other works on the subject, and has "run down" in health. He has tried different forms of material treatment, and wishes to avail himself of what may be found in the several forms of Occult Therapeutics. He finds himself offered several forms of occult healing. We will try to make plain to you how these different forms of healing operate, and the explanation behind each. We cannot give you detailed information and methods in a lesson of this size, for each system would require a volume to do that, but we hope to give you a general idea of the several forms of treatment.

MAGNETIC HEALING.

This is a form of Pranic Healing in which either the sick person or some "healer" sends an increased supply of Prana to the affected parts. Pranic healing really accompanies nearly every other form of healing, although its use is not suspected by those administering it. In what is known as "Magnetic Healing" the operator passes his hand over the body of the sick person, and by an effort of will, or strong desire, generates within himself a strong supply of Prana which he passes out to the patient. This

Prana acts as would a supply sent from the system
of the patient himself, and tends to strengthen and
invigorate the afflicted part of the body and to cause
it to function normally. In Magnetic Healing the
hands are usually passed over the body, the actual
touch usually being employed. We have given general directions regarding this form of healing in
"Science of Breath," and may, some day, issue a little
manual on the subject, giving specific directions.
We will give some general directions at the close of
this lesson, if space permits. We have said so much
about Prana in previous lessons, and in "Science of
Breath" that the student should be able to understand the principle behind this form of healing,
without much more explanation.

MENTAL HEALING.

Mental Healing covers a great deal of ground,
and has a number of apparently differing forms.
There is a form of Self-Healing which consists of
the repetitions of affirmations, or auto-suggestions,
by the patient, which tends to create a more cheerful and uplifting mental attitude, which reacts upon
the body and enables it to function properly. We
would say right here that the principal benefit de-
rived from this and kindred forms of healing lies in
the fact that it compels the patient to "let go" of adverse thoughts which have prevented Nature from
doing its work, rather than in any special virtue of
the affirmations. We have been refusing to let the
Divine Life Principle work freely through us, and

have hampered it with adverse auto-suggestion.
When we change our mental attitude we cease to
interpose this obstacle, and Nature soon reasserts
herself. Vigorous auto-suggestion, of course, stimulates the system and spurs up the Instinctive Mind
to its work.

In the form of mental treatment known as "Suggestion" the same principle operates. The mind of
the patient is relieved of adverse auto-suggestions
by the positive suggestions of the healer, and the
brake is taken off of the Instinctive Mind and Nature soon re-asserts herself, and a sufficient supply
of Prana is sent to the parts and soon a normal condition of affairs is re-established. In Suggestive
Treatment the healer usually, although often unconsciously, sends forth to the patient a supply of
his own Prana which stimulates the parts to action
and which renders easier the efforts of the patient's
mind to re-establish normal Pranic conditions.

In what is ordinarily known as "Mental Healing"
there is generally a considerable amount of suggestion used, although the healer may not be aware of
it. The mental attitude of the healer is impressed
upon the patient by the attitude, words, tone, and
demeanor of the healer, and the mind taking upon
the suggestion is benefited thereby. But, besides
this, the healer is pouring into the minds of the
patient a strong current of uplifting, strengthening,
and invigorating thought, which the patient receives
telepathically, particularly as a receptive mental attitude is manifested. The joining together of the

two minds in a common purpose produces a greatly increased directive force, and besides the mind of the patient being turned away from negative thoughts, a greater supply of Prana is absorbed and distributed through the body. The best form of Mental Treatment benefits both the mind and the body of the patient.

What is known as "Absent Mental Treatment" acts along precisely the same lines as the above mentioned form of Mental Treatment—the distance between patient and healer proving no obstacle to a strong healing thought. In both cases the healer often creates a powerful thought form, fully charged with Prana, which often produces an almost immediate effect upon the patient, the parts being greatly stimulated and strengthened. Instantaneous cures have often been made in this way, although comparatively few healers are sufficiently advanced to send thought-forms of this kind. A very powerful mental healer may be able to send a thought so highly charged with Prana, and so full of vital force and life, that a diseased organ may be filled with such recuperative force that it will begin instantly to cast off the waste and diseased matter and draw from the blood the elements necessary to rebuild and repair itself in a comparatively short space of time, in which case when the organism of the individual once re-establishes normal functioning the system is able to carry on the work without further help from outside.

All forms of Mental Healing come under one or

more of the above heads. Remember, now, the important point is to get the mind of the patient into
the proper mental attitude, casting out all forms of
adverse auto-suggestion, so that it will allow Nature
to do its work properly without interference. In
the process of accomplishing this result, the patient
may be aided (as above explained) by strong
thought directed to the afflicted part, and also by
sending a supply of Prana from the healer to stimulate the part and thus render easier the healing
work of the mind.

SPIRITUAL HEALING.

There is another form of healing, very rarely observed, in which a highly developed spiritual person
is able to let his spiritual aura and essence so de
scend upon an afflicted person that the entire system
becomes filled with it temporarily, and all abnor-
mality disappears, as Spirit being perfect transforms
all that with which it comes in contact. This true
Spiritual Healing is, however, so rare that very few
persons have had the good fortune to witness it. It
is claimed by many who are doing good work healing on other lines, but many of these persons are
self-deceived, and have not the faintest conception
of what true Spiritual Healing is. Spiritual Healing is marked by the *immediate* and *perfect* healing
of the patient, and the restoration of absolutely normal physical conditions, the patient being trans-
formed, physically, into a condition resembling that
of a robust, perfectly healthy, strong, vigorous child,

without a blemish, pain, particle of inharmony, or symptom of any kind. A few gifted individuals in the world in each age possess this power, but it is rarely manifested, for good occult reasons. And (draw a pencil line under these words) *true Spiritual Healing is never performed as a means of obtaining financial gain*—it is given "without money and without price." True Spiritual Healing is never tarnished by the slime of materiality—never! It is right and proper for "healers" to charge for Mental Healing and Pranic Healing in all forms, as they devote their time to the work, and "the laborer is worthy of his hire," and no desire is entertained to criticize such charges—they sell their services just as we sell these lessons, and are entitled to their just remuneration just as we are. But the individual who is able to give the real gift of Spiritual Healing is never placed in a position in which he finds it necessary to charge for his services—he is fed by the ravens, and has no need of bartering his spiritual gifts, and would die before he would so prostitute his divine privilege. We do not wish to be misunderstood in this matter—when we speak of Spiritual Healing we mean the true gifts of the Spirit, not some of the forms of Psychic or Mental healing miscalled "spiritual." If you would have an example of *true* Spiritual Healing, turn to the New Testament and read of the work of the Spirit as manifested through the Son of Mary. Let that be the standard—as in fact it is.

EXPERIMENTAL HEALING.

We find, to our satisfaction, that we will have suf-ficient space in which to give our students a few brief experiments in actual Occult Healing which they may practice. These experiments are given merely as examples, of course, and are not to be taken as being full instructions in the various forms of Occult Healing.

We will first take up a few experiments in Pranic Healing (or "Magnetic Healing," if you prefer the term):

(I) Let the patient sit in a chair, you standing before him. Let your hands hang loosely by your sides, and then swing them loosely to and fro for a few seconds, until you feel a tingling sensation at the tips of your fingers. Then raise them to the level of the patient's head, and sweep them slowly toward his feet, with your palms toward him with fingers outstretched, as if you were pouring force from your finger tips upon him. Then step back a foot and bring up your hands to the level of his head, being sure that your palms face each other in the upward movement, as, if you bring them up in the same position as you swept them down, you would draw back the magnetism you send toward him. Then repeat several times. In sweeping downward, do not stiffen the muscles, but allow the arms and hands to be loose and relaxed. You may treat the affected parts of the body in a similar way, finishing the treatment by saturating the entire body with magnetism. After treating the affected parts, it will be better for you to flick the fingers away from your sides, as if you were throwing off drops of water which had adhered to your fingers. Otherwise you might absorb some of the patient's conditions. This treatment is very strengthening to the patient, and if frequently practiced will greatly benefit him.

In case of chronic or long seated troubles, the trouble may often be "loosened up" by making "sideways" passes before the afflicted part, that is by standing before the patient with your hands together, palms touching, and then swinging the arms out sideways several times. This treatment should always be followed by the downward passes to equalize the circulation.

(II) In Chapter XIV, "Science of Breath," we have given a number of valuable experiments in this form of healing, which we advise the student to study and practice, if he is interested in this phase of the subject.

(III) Headaches may be relieved by having the patient sit down in front of you, you standing back of his chair, and passing your hands, fingers down and spread open in double circles over the top of his head, not touching his head, however. After a few seconds you will actually feel the passage of the magnetism from your fingers, and the patient's pain will be soothed.

(IV) Another good method of removing pain in the body is to stand before the patient, and present your palm to the affected part, at a distance of sev-

eral inches from the body. Hold the palm steady
for a few seconds and then begin a slow rotary motion, round and round, over the seat of the pain.
This is quite stimulating and tends to restore normal conditions.

(V) Point your forefinger toward the affected
part a few inches away from the body, and keeping
the finger steadily pointed move the hand around
just as if you were boring a hole with the point of
the finger. This will often start the circulation at
the point affected, and bring about improved conditions.

(VI) Placing the hands on the head of the patient, over the temples and holding them for a time,
has a good effect, and is a favorite form of treatment
of this kind.

(VII) Stroking the patient's body (over the
clothing) has a tendency to stimulate and equalize
the circulation, and to relieve congestion.

(VIII) Much of the value of Massage and similar forms of manipulative treatment, comes from
the Prana which is projected from the healer into
the patient, during the process of rubbing and manipulating. If the rubbing and manipulating is
accompanied by the conscious desire of the healer
to direct the flow of Prana into the patient a greatly
increased flow is obtained. If the practice is accompanied with Rhythmic Breathing, as explained in
"Science of Breath," the effect is much better.

(IX) Breathing upon the affected part, is practiced by many races of people, and is often a potent

means of conveying Prana to the affected part. This is often performed by placing a bit of cotton cloth between the flesh of the person and the healer, the breath heating up the cloth and adding the stimulation of warmth in addition to the other effects.

(X) Magnetized water is often employed by "magnetic healers", and many good results are reported to have been obtained in this way. The simplest form of magnetizing water is to hold the glass by the bottom, in the left hand, and then, gathering together the fingers of the right hand, shake them gently over the glass of water just as if you were shaking drops of water into the glass from your finger tips. You may add to the effect by afterwards making downward passes over the glass with the right hand, passing the Prana into the water. Rhythmic breathing will assist in the transferring of the Prana into the water. Water thus charged with Prana is stimulating to sick people, or those suffering from weakness, particularly if they sip it slowly holding their mind in a receptive attitude, and if possible forming a mental picture of the Prana from the water being taken up by the system and invigorating them.

We will now take up a few experiments in the several forms of Mental Healing, or Psychic Healing as some prefer to term it:

(I) Auto-suggestion consists in suggesting to oneself the physical conditions one wishes to bring about. The auto-suggestions should be spoken (audibly or silently) just as one would speak to

another, earnestly and seriously, letting the mind
form a mental picture of the conditions referred to
in the words. For instance: *"My stomach is strong,
strong, strong—able to digest the food given it—able
to assimilate the nourishment from the food—able
to give me the nourishment which means health
and strength to me. My digestion is good, good,
good, and I am enjoying and digesting and assimilating my food, converting it into rich red blood,
which is carrying health and strength to all parts of
my body, building it up and making me a strong
man (or woman)."* Similar auto-suggestions, or affirmations, applied to other parts of the body, will
work equally good results, the attention and mind
being directed to the parts mentioned causing an
increased supply of Prana to be sent there, and the
pictured condition to be brought about. Enter into
the spirit of the auto-suggestions, and get thoroughly
in earnest over them, and so far as possible form the
mental image of the healthy condition desired. See
yourself as you wish yourself to be. You may help
the cure along by treating yourself by the methods
described in the experiments on Pranic Healing.

(II) Suggestions of healing, given to others, operate on the same principle as do the auto-suggestions just described, except that the healer must
impress upon the mind of the patient the desired
conditions instead of the patient's doing it for himself. Much better results may be obtained where
the healer and patient both co-operate in the mental image and when the patient follows the healer's

suggestions in his mind, and forms the mental picture implied by the healer's words. The healer suggests that which he wishes to bring about and the patient allows the suggestions to sink into his Instinctive Mind, where they are taken up and afterwards manifested in physical results. The best suggestionists are men of vitality, who send forceful thoughts charged with Prana into the organism of the patient, at the same time that the suggestions are given. In nearly all forms of mental healing, several methods are intermingled, as the student will discover for himself, if he takes the trouble to analyze the treatments. The Instinctive Mind often falls into bad habits of attending to the body, by reason of the person having departed from the natural way of living and having caused the Instinctive Mind to take up these incorrect habits. Suggestion, and auto-suggestion bring back the Instinctive Mind to normal functioning, and the body speedily recovers its former harmony. In many cases all that is needed in suggestive treatment, is to relieve the patient's mind of Fear and Worry and depressing thoughts, which have interfered with the proper harmony of the body, and which have prevented the proper amount of Prana from being distributed to the parts. Removing these harmful thoughts is like removing the speck of dust which has caused our watch to run improperly, having disarranged the harmony of the delicate mechanism. Fear, Worry and Hate, with their accompanying emotions, are the cause of more physical inharmony than nearly all the other causes combined.

(III) In what is called strictly Mental Healing, the patient sits in a relaxed attitude of body, and allows the mind to become receptive. The healer then projects to the patient thoughts of a strengthening and uplifting character which, reacting upon the mind of the patient, causes it to cast off its negative conditions and to assume its normal poise and power, the result being that as soon as the patient's mind recovers its equilibrium it asserts itself and starts into operation the recuperative power within the organism of the person, sending an increased supply of Prana to all parts of the body and taking the first step toward regaining health and strength. The prime principle of Mental Healing is to get the *mind* of the patient into the proper condition, it naturally following that beneficial and normal physical conditions must follow. But the best Mental Healers do more than this—they (often unconsciously) send a positive thought strongly charged with Prana right to the affected spot, and actually work a physical change in the organism of the patient, independent of what is accomplished by his own thought-force. In treating a patient in this way, keep firmly in your mind the thought that physical harmony is being re-established in the patient, and that health is his normal condition and that all the negative thoughts are being expelled from his mind. Picture him as strong and healthy in mind and in body. Picture as existing all the conditions you wish to establish within him. Then concentrate the mind and fairly *dart* into his body, or into the affected part, a strong penetrating thought, the purpose of which is to work the desired physical change, casting out the abnormal conditions and re-establishing normal conditions and functioning. Form the mental image that the thought is fully and heavily charged with Prana, and fairly drive it into the affected part by an effort of the will. Considerable practice is usually needed to accomplish this last result, but to some it appears to come without much effort.

(IV) Distant healing, or "absent treatment," is performed in precisely the same way as is the treatment when the patient is present. We have given some directions regarding this form of treatment in Chapter XIV, "Science of Breath," which, coupled with what we have just said in the last paragraph, should give an elementary working knowledge of the subject. Some healers form the picture of the patient sitting in front of them, and then proceed to give the treatment, just as if the patient were really present. Others form the mental image of projecting the thought, picturing it as leaving their mind, and then traversing space entering the mind of the patient. Others merely sit in a passive, contemplative attitude and intently *think* of the patient, without regard to intervening space. Others prefer to have a handkerchief, or some other article belonging to the patient, in order to render more perfect the *rapport* conditions. Any, or all, of these methods are good, the temperament and inclinations of the person causing him to prefer some particular method. But the same principle underlies them all.

A little practice along the lines of the several forms of healing just mentioned, will give the student confidence, and ease in operating the healing power, until he will often radiate healing power without being fully conscious of it. If much healing work is done, and the heart of the healer is in his work, he soon gets so that he heals almost automatically and involuntarily when he comes into the presence of one who is suffering. The healer must, however, guard against depleting himself of Prana, and thus injuring his own health. He should study up the methods given by us, of recharging himself, and protecting himself against undue drains upon his vitality. And he should make haste slowly in these matters, remembering that forced growth is not desirable.

This lesson has not been written for the purpose of advising our students to become healers. They must use their own judgment and intuitions regarding that question. We have devoted the lesson to the subject, as it formed a part of the general subject which we are treating in this course, and it is important that they should know something of the principles underlying these several forms of healing. Let them analyze any form of treatment which they may witness or hear of, stripping it of all the fantastic theories which have been built around it, and they will be able to classify and study it without accepting the theory of the person making the cure.

Remember that *all* the cults and schools make cures, using the same principle, but attributing the result to widely differing theories and beliefs.

For ourselves, we cling to the principles of "Hatha Yoga," which teaches the doctrine of preserving health by right living and right thinking, and we regard all forms of healing as things made necessary only by Man's ignorance and disobedience of Natural laws. But so long as man will not live and think properly, some forms of healing are necessary, and therefore the importance of their study. The advanced occultist regards the preservation of health as a more important thing for the race than the cure of disease, believing with the old adage, that "an ounce of prevention is worth a pound of cure." But so long as we may benefit our fellow men, it is well that we know something of the subject of Occult Therapeutics. It is one of Nature's forces, and we should know how to use it.

THE NINTH LESSON.

PSYCHIC INFLUENCE.

One of the things which have puzzled scientific investigators and students of the history of mankind is the persistent recurrence of stories, legends and traditions relating to the possession and practice of some form of Psychic Influence by men of all races and in all ages. The investigators have found it easy to dismiss the more primitive forms of these stories by the explanation that they were merely the result of the crudest form of superstition among the uneducated and undeveloped people. But as they turned over the pages of history they found that the "idle superstition" still maintained its original force, and that its forms increased in number and variety. From the repulsive Voodoo practices of the African savage, one may trace a straight line to the Witch-craft epidemic in New England, and thence on to the present time, when the Western world has apparently gone wild on "psychism," and the daily papers are filled with sensational tales of mesmeric influence, hypnotism, personal magnetism, etc. The books of all ages are filled with tales of psychic influence, the Bible containing a number of instances of its practice for good or evil.

165

At the present time, attention is often called to the wonderful instances of the power of the mind, personal magnetism, etc., and it is quite common to hear the expression that one has, or has not, "personal magnetism"—is, or is not, "magnetic." Much nonsense has been written on this subject, and some of the wildest assertions and theories regarding it have been advanced. And yet, the truth itself is far more wonderful than are the wildest fictions which have been written and taught regarding it. Underlying all the popular notions and misconceptions regarding Psychic Influence lies a solid basis of fact, the greater portion of which is undreamt of by even many of those who have been feeding the public taste for sensationalism.

We need scarcely tell our students that the Orientals have known and practiced, for centuries past, all known forms of occultism, and, in fact, have possessed the secrets which the investigators of the West have been striving so laboriously to uncover. Scraps of the knowledge have filtered through, and have been eagerly seized upon by Western writers, and used as the basis for startling claims and theories.

And, much of this hidden knowledge will, and must, remain hidden for years to come, because of the undeveloped state of the race and the general unfitness of people for this secret wisdom. To spread before the general public even a small part of certain of the hidden teachings, at this time, would be dangerous indeed, and would bring upon the race one of the greatest curses known to man. This not because of any wrong in the teachings themselves, but because the selfishness of the average man or woman is such that they would soon begin to use this knowledge for their own personal profit and ends, to the detriment and hurt of their fellow-men. This would avail them nothing if the entire race knew enough of the subject—had advanced far enough intellectually and spiritually to grasp and comprehend these teachings, and thus be able to protect themselves from the selfish attempts of their unscrupulous brothers and sisters. For, as all occultists know, no Black Magic can affect the man or woman who knows his or her real place in nature— his or her real powers to resist the practices of those who have acquired bits of occult knowledge without the spiritual growth which would teach them how to use same properly. But the average person of to-day does not know—and will not be convinced —of his own power, and therefore is unable to protect himself from the psychic attempts of even those who have grasped some fragments of occult teachings, and are using them for selfish ends.

The improper use of psychic power has long been known to occultists as "Black Magic," which, so far from being a remnant of the superstition of the Middle Ages, is a very real thing, and is being practiced to-day to a great extent. Those so practicing it are sowing the seeds of their own punishment, and every bit of psychic force expended for base and selfish ends will unquestionably rebound and react upon the user, but nevertheless these people are influencing others that they may reap some material gain or pleasure, and the public is being more or less imposed upon by such people, although it laughs at the idea—considers the matter a joke—and regards those who teach the truth as wild visionaries or mentally weak.

Very fortunately, those who would so prostitute psychic powers know comparatively little regarding the subject, and can use only the simpler forms, but when they come in contact with those entirely ignorant of the subject, they are able to accomplish more or less by their arts. Many men find, sometimes by accident, that they can influence others to their bidding, and not knowing the source of their power often use it just as they would any physical power, or mental strength. Such people, however, usually have gradually brought to their knowledge (in pursuance with well-established occult laws) something which will lead them to a better understanding of the subject, and they begin to see their mistake. Others pick up a little bit of occult teaching, and "try it on" others, and, seeing the effect, start on the road to "Black Magic," although scarcely knowing what they are doing. These people, also, are warned in certain ways, and given every chance to rectify their error. Others seem to understand something of the risk they are running, but willingly take it, being fascinated by their new sense of power, and blinded by it.

None of these people are allowed to go very far with their selfish work, as there are certain influences at work to counteract their efforts, and a little good always counteracts a great deal of the selfish psychic work—this being an old occult truth.

But outside of this bit of elementary "Black Magic," of which we have spoken more in the way of a warning and a caution, many people are endowed with faculties which make them powers among their fellow-men and women, and their influence is felt in every-day life, just as the influence of the physically strong man is felt in a crowd of weaker people. It needs but a moment's glance at one's acquaintances to show that some of them have a greater influence than have others. Some are naturally looked to as leaders and teachers, while others naturally fall into place as followers. These strong, positive men come to the front in warfare, business life, the bar, the pulpit, in the practice of medicine, and in fact, in all walks of life and all branches of human endeavor. We notice this fact, and speak of this man being possessed of a great deal of "Personal Magnetism," or of that one lacking it. But what do we mean by "Personal Magnetism"? Can anyone give an intelligent answer? Many are the theories which have been advanced to account for this phenomenon, and many are the plans advanced to develop this "power." Of late years many teachers have sprung up, claiming to have discovered this secret and offering to teach it to all comers at so many dollars a head, many sensational announcements having been made to attract purchasers of "courses" of instruction, and many appeals to the most selfish motives have been made in order to awaken an interest in what is offered for sale. In the majority of cases these teachers have practically nothing to offer and teach, while in some few cases they have worked out a sufficient knowledge of the subject to be able to give directions whereby one may possess himself of a sufficient degree of psychic power to gain a certain amount of influence over the ignorant and weak of the race. But, fortunately, the majority of these purchasers of these teachings have not sufficient confidence in themselves or in the teachings to put into practice even the compara-tively meagre teachings given them. But at least a few have sufficient self-confidence to put these plans into practice, and are able to do considerable harm by their ignorant and selfish use of powers which are intended for high uses. All these things must pass away as the race advances in knowledge and understanding of the occult truths, and, in the mean-time, those who really understand the subject are doing what they can to educate the race in its prin-ciples, that they may protect themselves, psychically, and may not be tempted to make a selfish use of the higher powers.

The man or woman of spiritual growth and de-velopment can afford to smile at the efforts of these dabblers in "Black Magic," at least so far as the fear of any personal injury to or effect upon themselves is concerned. Such a one rises to a higher plane to which the efforts of the selfish occultist (?) cannot penetrate. We will have something to say on this subject of Self Protection, toward the end of this lesson, after we have given the student a general idea of the several forms of Psychic Influence in general use.

We wish to be distinctly understood, however, when we say that no attempt will be made in this lesson to uncover a degree of occult knowledge which might place in the hands of the chance reader a weapon to use for his own selfish ends. This is a lesson designed for the Self Protection of those who read it—not for the advancement of a knowledge of "Black Magic" even in its elementary forms. And let us here caution those who read what we will write on this subject that we are serious in what we say regarding the selfish use of occult knowledge—if they knew but a fragment of the trouble which one may bring upon himself by improper occult practices, they would drop the subject as quickly as they would a venomous serpent which was beginning to warm into life from the heat of their hands. Occult powers are for the proper use and protection of mankind, not for misuse or abuse, and, like playing with the wires of a dynamo, meddling with these powers is apt to prove unpleasant to the person who will not heed the warning.

Although many Western writers deny it, all true occultists know that all forms of Psychic Influence, including what is called "Personal Magnetism," "Mesmerism," "Hypnotism," "Suggestion," etc., are but different manifestations of the same thing. What this "thing" is may be readily imagined by those who have followed us in our preceding lessons. It is the power of the Mind of the individual, operated along the lines mentioned in our preceding lessons. We trust that the student has acquainted himself with what we have said regarding "The Instinctive Mind," "Thought Dynamics," "Telepathy," "Thought Forms," etc., as well as the potency of Prana, that he may understand this lesson without too much repetition.

Psychic Influence—and by this we mean all forms of it—what does it mean? Of what does it consist? How is it called into operation? What is its effect? Let us try to answer these questions.

We must begin with the Instinctive Mind—one of the Seven Principles of Man. We told you (in Lesson II) that this is a plane of mentation shared in common with us by the lower animals, at least in its lowest forms. It is the first form of mentation reached in the scale of evolution, and, in its lowest stages manifests entirely along sub-conscious lines. Its beginnings are seen as far back as the mineral life, manifesting here in the formation of crystals, etc. In the lower forms of plant life it shows but feebly, and is scarcely a degree above that manifested by the mineral. Then, by easy and progressive stages it grows more distinct and higher in the scale, in plant life, until in some of the higher forms of plants it even manifests a rudimentary form of consciousness. In the kingdom of the lower animals, the Instinctive Mind is seen in varying stages, from the almost plant-like intelligence of the lowest forms of animal life to the almost human intelligence of some of the higher animals. Then in the lower forms of human life we find it scarcely removed from the highest form shown in the lower animals, and as we ascend in the scale we find it becoming shaded, colored, and influenced by the fifth principle, the Intellect, until we reach the highest form of man known to us at this time where we see the Intellect in control, asserting its proper position, and influencing the lower principle only for good, and avoiding the mistakes of the less developed man who pours harmful auto-suggestions into the Instinctive Mind, and works actual harm to himself.

In this consideration of the Instinctive Mind, we must pass over its wonderful work in superintending the work of the physical body, and also some of its other manifestations, and must confine ourselves to the subject of the part the Instinctive Mind plays in the matter of Psychic Influence—a most important part, by the way, as, without the Instinctive Mind there could be no operation of Psychic Influence, as there would be nothing to be acted upon. The Instinctive Mind is the instrument played upon by Psychic Influence. We speak, often, as if one's Intellect were influenced in this way, but this is incorrect, for the person is influenced *in spite* of his Intellect, not by means of it—the influence is so strongly impressed upon the Instinctive Mind that it runs away heedless of the protests of the Intellect, as many persons afterwards recollect to their sorrow.

Many are the persons who, in their own words, "knew better all the time, but did it just the same."

We will start with what is known as "Suggestion," and which really lies at the bottom of all forms of Psychic Influence, personal or "absent." By Suggestion we mean the influencing or control of the thoughts and actions of another by means of a positive command, or a subtle insinuation of the desired thought, or any combination of the two, or anything that may come between these two extremes. Personal Suggestion is quite common in everyday life, in fact, we are constantly giving and taking suggestions, consciously and unconsciously, and one can scarcely get away from the giving and taking, so long as he associates with other persons—hears their voices or reads what others have written or printed. But these everyday suggestions are relatively unimportant, and lack the force of a conscious and deliberate suggestion by one who understands the "Art of Suggesting." Let us first see how and why the suggestions are received and acted upon.

As we have said, in the early forms of life the Instinctive Mind worked on alone, uninfluenced by Intellect (for Intellect had not yet unfolded or developed) totally unconscious, as in plant life. As the scale of evolution was mounted, the animal began to become dimly conscious, and commenced to be "aware" of things, and to perform a something like primitive reasoning about them. In order to protect itself from its enemies, the animal had to be guided by the rudimentary consciousness which was beginning to unfold, and which manifested in and through the Instinctive Mind. Some animals progressed more rapidly than others of their kind, and naturally began to assert themselves and their peculiar power—they found themselves doing the thinking for their fellows. They came to be recognized as being the ones to look to in cases of danger, or when food became scarce, and their leading was generally recognized and followed. Leaders sprang up in flocks and herds, and not alone (as has been commonly taught in the text-books) because of their brute strength, but also because of their superior brain-power, which may be described as "cunning." The "cunning" animal was quick to recognize danger, and to take means to avoid it—quick to discover new ways to gain food, and overcome the common enemy, or the prey. Anyone who has been much around domestic animals—or who has studied the ways of the wild animals who flock together—will realize exactly what we mean. The few led and directed, and the many blindly followed and were led.

And, as the development went on, and Man was evolved, the same thing manifested itself—leaders sprang into prominence and were obeyed. And all along the history of the race up until the present time, this same state of affairs exists. A few lead and the many follow. Man is an obedient and imitative animal. The great majority of people are like sheep—give them a "bell-wether" and they will gladly follow the tinkle of the bell.

But mark this fact—it is a most important one—it

is not always the man or woman of the greatest amount of what we call "intellectual attainment," education or "book-learning" who is the leader of men—on the contrary, many of such people are often the most confirmed followers of leaders. The man or woman who leads is the one who feels within himself, or herself, that something which may be called a consciousness of power—an awareness of the real source of strength and power behind them and in them. This "awareness" may not be recognized by the Intellect, it may not be understood, but the individual *feels* somehow that he is possessed of power and force, or is in contact with power and force which he may use. And (speaking of the ordinary man) he consequently gives himself a personal credit for it, and begins to use his power. He feels the reality of the word "I." He feels himself as an individual—a real thing—an entity—and he, instinctively, proceeds to assert himself. These people, as a rule, do not understand the source of their power, but it is a matter of "feeling" with them, and they naturally make use of the power. They influence others, without understanding just "how," and often wonder how it all comes about. And how *does* it come about? Let us see.

Let us look to the persons who are influenced. What part of their mental mechanism or armament is affected? The Instinctive Mind, of course. And why are their Instinctive Minds affected so easily, while others are so much less so? That's just the point; let us look into the matter.

In the original state, and during the process of evolution, the Instinctive Mind was not influenced thusly, *because there was nothing to influence it.* But as Man developed, the individuals who became aware of the dawning sense of their "individuality" and real power, began to assert themselves, and their own Instinctive Minds and the Instinctive Minds of others began to be influenced. The man whose consciousness of individuality—whose awareness of the "I"—is largely developed, invariably influences the Instinctive Mind of the one in whom the consciousness is not so fully developed. The Instinctive Mind of the less conscious man takes up and acts upon the suggestions of the stronger "I," and also allows the latter's thought-waves to beat upon it and to be absorbed.

Remember, once more, that it is not the man of purely intellectual attainment, culture, or "learning" who has this consciousness, although, of course, the higher the intellectual attainment of the man the greater the scope of the power of the conscious "I" he may possess. Uneducated men are seen to have this power, as well as the most highly educated, and although their deficient education and training prevents them making use of their power to the extent possible to their more favored brother, still they exert an influence upon all in their "class," and also upon many who have greater intellectual powers than have they. It is not a matter of education, or of abstract reasoning, etc.—*it is a matter of "consciousness."* Those who possess it somehow

feel the "I" within them, and although it often leads
one to an absurd degree of egotism, vain self-pride
and conceit, yet a man possessing this consciousness
to any extent invariably influences others and forces
his way through the world. The world has given to
this manifestation of this consciousness the name of
"self-confidence," etc. You will readily recognize
it, if you think a moment and look around you a
little. There are, of course, many degrees of this
consciousness, and, everything else being equal, the
man or woman will exert an influence upon others
in precisely the degree that they possess this power.
This consciousness may be developed and increased.
It is, however, inferior to the consciousness of the
man or woman of spiritual attainment, or development, whose powers greatly exceed this consciousness on the mental plane.

But to get back to our subject of *how* the Instinctive Mind is influenced. The man whose consciousness of "I" is sufficiently developed, suggests to his
own Instinctive Mind, and the latter naturally looks
to its master as the only source of command or instruction. But the one who has not this consciousness has given but feeble commands of this kind,
and his Instinctive Mind is not instilled with that
confidence that it should possess, and finds its master
frequently (often invariably) allowing it to receive
the commands and instructions of others, until it
automatically takes up and acts upon almost any
forcible suggestion coming from without. Such
outside suggestions may be either verbal sugges-

tions or suggestions conveyed by the thought-waves of others.

Many people have no confidence whatever in their own "I"—they are like human sheep, and naturally follow their leader—in fact, are unhappy unless they are led. The more forcible the commands, the more ready they are to obey. Any statement made to them positively and authoritatively is accepted and acted upon. Such people live upon "authority," and constantly seek for "precedents" and "examples"—they need somebody to lean upon.

To sum up the matter—they are mentally lazy so far as exercising the "I" consciousness and developing the same is concerned—and they consequently have not asserted their control over their Instinctive Mind, but allow it to be open to the suggestions and influence of others, who, very often, are less qualified to direct it than they are themselves, but who happen to have a little more "self-confidence" and "assurance"—a little more consciousness of the "I."

Now as to the means whereby the Instinctive Mind is influenced. There are innumerable methods and forms of practices, conscious and unconscious, whereby such effects are produced, but they may be roughly grouped into three general classes, viz. (1) Personal Suggestion; (2) Thought Influence, present and distant, and (3) Mesmeric or Hypnotic Influence. These three forms shade into each other, and are generally combined, but it is well to separate them here, that we may understand them the better. We will take them up in turn, briefly.

Let us first consider Personal Suggestion. As we have said, this is most common, and is constantly practiced more or less by all of us, and we are all more or less affected by it. We will confine ourselves to the most striking forms. Personal Suggestions are conveyed by the voice, the manner, the appearance, etc. The Instinctive Mind takes for granted, and accepts as truth the words, appearance and manners of the positive person, and acts upon the same, according to degree of its receptivity. This degree varies in persons, according to the degree to which they have developed the "I" consciousness, as we have before stated. The greater the amount of the "I" consciousness, the less the degree of receptivity, unless the person is tired, his attention is distracted, is off his guard, or voluntarily opens himself to the influence of the other's mind or words.

The more positive or authoritative the suggestion the more readily is it taken up by the receptive Instinctive Mind. Suggestion affects a person not through his Intellect but through his Instinctive Mind—it operates not by argument but by assertions, demands and commands. Suggestions gain force by being repeated, and where one is not influenced by a single suggestion, repeated suggestions along the same lines have a much greater power. Some persons have cultivated such a proficiency in the art of Suggestion that one has to be on his guard not to unconsciously accept some of the subtle suggestions insinuated into the conversation. But one who realizes the "I" consciousness, or, better still, the Real Self and its relation to All, has no need to fear the power of the suggestionist, as the suggestions will not be able to penetrate his well-guarded Instinctive Mind, or even if it does lodge around the outer surface of the mind, it will soon be detected and discarded with a smile of amusement. But, a word of caution; be on your guard towards those who attempt to lead you not by argument or reason, but by assertion, pretended authority, plausible manner and a general "taking it for granted" way with you. Also keep your eye on those who ask you questions and answer them in advance for you, thus: "You like this pattern, don't you?" or "This is what you want, isn't it?" Suggestion and assertion go hand in hand. You can generally tell a Suggestion by the company it keeps.

Secondly, let us consider Thought Influence, present and distant. As we have stated in previous lessons, every thought results in the projection of thought-waves of greater or lesser strength, size and power. We have explained how these thought-waves are sent forth, and how they are received by another individual. We are all receiving thought-waves at all times, but comparatively few affect us, as they are not in harmony with our own thoughts, moods, character and tastes. We attract to our inner consciousness only such thoughts as are in harmony with our own. But, if we are of a negative character, and allow our Instinctive Mind to go without its proper master, and become too receptive, we are in danger of having it accept, assimilate and act upon the passing thought-waves surrounding us. We have explained the action of the thought-waves in other lessons, but we did not point out this phase of the matter, preferring to take it up here. The unguarded Instinctive Mind is not only affected by all sorts of passing thought-waves, which are floated down to it, but is also peculiarly liable to be affected by a strong, positive, conscious thought-wave directed toward it by another who wishes to influence its owner. Everyone who is trying to influence another person, for good or evil, unconsciously throws off thought-waves of this kind with greater or less effect. And some who have learned some of the rudimentary occult truths and have prostituted them into Black Magic, consciously and deliberately send thought-waves towards persons whom they wish to influence. And if the Instinctive Mind is unguarded by its proper master, it is more or less apt to be affected by these efforts of selfish and malicious minds.

The tales of Witchcraft days are not all mere delusions and superstitions, but underneath the exaggerated reports and tales may be found a great foundation of occult truth, readily recognized by the advanced occultist as rudimentary occult power prostituted into Black Magic. All the combined Black Magic or Witchcraft in the world could not affect a man or woman who possessed the higher form of consciousness, but one of a fearful, superstitious turn of mind, with little or no self-confidence or self-reliance, would be apt to have an Instinctive Mind ready and ripe for the entrance of such hurtful thought-waves or thought-forms. All the conjurations, "spells," etc., of the voodoos, "witches," conjurers, etc., etc., have no efficacy beyond the thought sent out with their use—and the thought is made more powerful because it is concentrated by means of the rites, ceremonies, "spells," images, etc., of the unholy devotees of Black Magic. But it would be just as powerful if concentrated by some other means. But, no matter how concentrated or sent forth, it can have no effect unless the Instinctive Mind is ready to receive and assimilate it, and act upon it. The man or woman "who knows" need have no fear of these practices. In fact, the very reading of this lesson will clear away from many minds the receptivity which might have, or has had, allowed them to be influenced to a greater or lesser extent by the selfish thoughts of others. This, mind you, not because of any virtue in this lesson (we are claiming nothing of the sort), but merely because the reading of it has caused the student's mind to awaken to its own power, and to assert itself.

Remember, the mind attracts only such thoughts as are harmonious with its own thoughts—and the Instinctive Mind is influenced against its own interests, only when its owner has admitted his own weakness and lack of ability to master and guard it. You must guard your own Instinctive Mind, and assert your master and ownership of it, as, otherwise, that ownership may be asserted, claimed and usurped by others more masterful than yourself. You have the strength and power necessary within you, if you but assert it. It is yours for the asking— why don't you demand it? You may awaken the "I" consciousness and develop it by the power of assertion, which will aid in its unfoldment. We will have more to say on this point in the following pages.

We will now consider the third form of Psychic Influence, which is known as Mesmerism, Hypnotism, etc. We can merely touch upon that subject here, as its varied forms and phenomena would fill books, if spread out. But we think we can make it clear to you in a few words, as you have followed our thoughts in this and the preceding lessons.

The first thing to remember is that Mesmerism or Hypnotism is but a combination of the two methods just mentioned, plus a greater amount of Prana projected with the Personal Suggestion or Thought-Wave. In other words, the Suggestion or Thought-Wave becomes charged with Prana to a greater degree than is ordinarily the case, and becomes as much stronger than the ordinary suggestion or thought-wave, as a thought-form is stronger than an ordinary thought-wave. In short, mesmerism or hypnotism is practically the bathing of the person in a flow of thought-forms, kept stimulated and active by a constant supply of Prana, which has in such cases often been called "the mesmeric fluid."

And, another thing to remember is that no person can be mesmerized or hypnotised unless his Instinctive Mind is unguarded or without its proper master, unless the person agrees to be mesmerized and actually consents to it. So that, in the end, it comes down to the fact that no person need be mesmerized or hypnotised unless he is willing or unless he believes that he may be, which is the same thing in the end. Mesmerism has its uses in the hands of the advanced occultist who understands its laws, but in the hands of those ignorant of its proper use it is a thing to be avoided. Be careful about allowing yourself to be hypnotised by the ignorant pretender. Assert your own power, and you may accomplish for yourself all that anyone else can, on the same plane.

We have, in the brief space at our disposal, touched upon the various forms of Psychic Influence, and may have an opportunity at some future time of going deeper into the subject with you. But we trust that we have said enough to give you at least a general knowledge of the subject, and have at the same time given you a timely warning and caution. We will conclude by saying something to you about the "I" consciousness and its development, which we trust you will read with the attention it merits, and will put into practice that which is indicated.

There is, of course, a still higher form of consciousness than the "I" consciousness—the spiritual consciousness which causes one to be aware of his relation to, and connection with, the source of all power. And those possessing this higher consciousness are far beyond the influence of Psychic Influence of others, for they are surrounded with an aura which repels vibrations on a lower plane. Such do not need the "I" consciousness, as it is included in their higher consciousness. But those on the mental plane of development (and but few of us have progressed further) will find it well to develop and unfold their consciousness of the "I"—the sense of individuality. You will be aided in this by carrying in mind, and meditating often, that you are a real thing—that you are an Ego—a bit of the Universal Life set apart as an individual that you may work out your part of the Universal Plan, and progress to higher forms of manifestation. That YOU are independent of the body, and only use same as an instrument—that YOU are indestructible, and have eternal life—that YOU cannot be destroyed by fire, water or anything else which the physical man looks upon as a thing which will "kill" him—that no matter what becomes of your body YOU will survive. YOU are a soul, and have a body. (Not that you are a body having a soul, as most persons think and act upon.) Think of yourself as an independent being, using the body as a convenience. Cultivate the feeling of immortality and reality, and you will gradually begin to realize that you really exist and will always exist, and Fear will drop from you like a discarded cloak, for Fear is really the thought weakening the ill-guarded Instinctive Mind—once get rid of Fear, and the rest is easy. We have spoken of this matter in "Science of Breath," under the title of "Soul Consciousness," on page 70. In the same book, on page 61, under the title "Forming an Aura," we have hinted at a plan whereby weak and fearful persons may protect themselves while they are building up a sure foundation of self-confidence and strength. The affirmation or mantram which has proven of more benefit than any other in these cases is the positive assertion of "I AM," which expresses a truth and tends to a mental attitude which is taken up by the Instinctive Mind and renders it more positive to others, and less liable to be affected by suggestions, etc. The mental attitude expressed by "I AM" will surround you with a thought aura, which will act as a shield and a protection, until such time as you have fully acquired the higher consciousness, which carries with it a sense of self-confidence and assurance of strength.

From this point you will gradually develop into that consciousness which assures you that when you say "I," you do not speak only of the individual entity, with all its strength and power, but know that the "I" has behind it the power and strength of the Spirit, and is connected with an inexhaustible supply of force, which may be drawn upon when needed. Such a one can never experience Fear—for he has risen far above it. Fear is the manifestation of weakness, and so long as we hug it to us and make a bosom friend of it, we will be open to the influences of others. But by casting aside Fear we take several steps upward in the scale, and place ourselves in touch with the strong, helpful, fearless, courageous thought of the world, and leave behind us all the old weaknesses and troubles of the old life.

When man learns that nothing can really harm him, Fear seems a folly. And when man awakens to a realization of his real nature and destiny, he knows that nothing can harm him, and consequently Fear is discarded.

It has been well said, "There is nothing to fear, but Fear," and in this epigram is concealed a truth which all advanced occultists will recognize. The abolishing of Fear places in the hands of Man a weapon of defense and power which renders him almost invincible. Why do you not take this gift which is so freely offered you? Let your watchwords be: " I AM." "I AM FEARLESS AND FREE."

THE TENTH LESSON.

THE ASTRAL WORLD.

We are confronted with a serious difficulty at the beginning of this lesson, which will be apparent to those of our students who are well advanced in occult studies. We allude to the matter of the description of "planes" of existence. These lessons are intended as elementary studies designed to give the beginner a plain, simple idea of the general principles of occultism, without attempting to lead him into the more complicated stages of the subject. We have tried to avoid technicalities, so far as is possible, and believe that we have at least fairly well accomplished our task of presenting elementary principles in a plain manner, and we know that we have succeeded in interesting many persons in the study, who had heretofore been deterred from taking it up because of the mass of technical description and complicated description of details that met their view upon taking up other works on the subject.

So, in this lesson on the Astral World, and the three lessons that follow it, we will be compelled to deal in generalities instead of going into minute and careful descriptions such as would be needed in

a work taking up the "higher-grade" work. Instead
of endeavoring to describe just what a "plane" is,
and then going on to point out the nice little differences between "planes" and "sub-planes" we shall
treat the whole subject of the higher planes of existence under the general term of "The Astral World,"
making that term include not only the lower divisions of the Astral Plane, but also some of the
higher planes of life. This plan may be objected to
by some who have followed other courses of reading on the subject, in which only the lower Astral
Plane has been so styled, the higher planes receiving
other names, which has led many to regard the
Astral Plane with but scanty consideration reserv-
ing their careful study for the higher planes. But
we ask these persons to remember that many of the
ancient occultists classed the entire group of the
upper planes (at least until the higher spiritual
planes were reached) under the general term "The
Astral World," or similar terms, and we have the
best of authority for this general division. There is
as much difference between the lowest astral planes
and the highest mental or spiritual planes, as there
is between a gorilla and an Emerson, but in order
to keep the beginner from getting lost in a wilder-
ness of terms, we have treated all the planes above
the physical (at least such as our lessons touches
upon) under the general style of "The Astral
World."

It is difficult to convey clearly, in simple terms,
the meaning of the word "plane," and we shall use

it but little, preferring the word "state," for a plane is really a "state" rather than a place—that is, any one place may be inhabited on several planes. Just as a room may be filled with rays of the sun; light from a lamp; rays from an X-ray apparatus; ordinary magnetic vibrations; air, etc., etc., each acting according to the law of its being, and yet not affecting the others, so may several planes of being be in full operation in a given space, without interfering with each other. We cannot go into detail regarding the matter, in this elementary lesson, and hope merely to give the student a good working mental conception, in order that he may understand the incidents and phenomena of the several planes comprising "The Astral World."

Before going into the subject of the several planes of the Astral World, it will be better for us to consider some of the general phenomena classified under the term "astral." In our Sixth Lesson, we have told you that man (in the body), in addition to his physical senses of sight, hearing, tasting, smelling and feeling, has five *astral* senses (counterparts of the physical senses) operating on the astral plane, by which he may receive sense impressions without the aid of the physical sense organs. He also possesses a "sixth-sense" physical organ (the organ of the "telepathic" sense) which also has a corresponding astral sense.

These astral senses function on the lower astral plane—the plane next removed from the physical plane—and the phenomena of clairvoyance is produced by the use of these astral senses, as we have described in the Sixth Lesson. There are, of course, higher forms of clairvoyance, which operate on planes far above that used in ordinary clairvoyance, but such powers are so rare, and are possessed only by those of high attainment, that we need scarcely do more than mention them here. On this lower astral plane, the clairvoyant sees; the clairaudient hears; the psychometrist feels. On this plane the astral body moves about, and "ghosts" manifest. Disembodied souls living on the higher planes of the Astral World, in order to communicate with those on the physical plane, must descend to this lowest plane, and clothe themselves with coarse astral matter in order to accomplish their object. On this plane moves the "astral bodies" of those in the flesh, who have acquired the art of projecting themselves in the astral. It is possible for a person to project his astral body, or travel in his astral body, to any point within the limits of the earth's attraction, and the trained occultist may do so at will, under the proper conditions. Others may occasionally take such trips (without knowing just how they do it, and having, afterwards, the remembrance of a particular and very vivid dream); in fact many of us do take such trips, when the physical body is wrapped in sleep, and one often gains much information in this way, upon subjects in which he is interested, by holding astral communication with others interested in the same subject, all unconsciously of course. The conscious acquirement of knowledge in this way, is possible only to those who have progressed quite a way along the path of attainment. The trained occultist merely places himself in the proper mental condition, and then wishes himself at some particular place, and his astral travels there with the rapidity of light, or even more rapidly. The untrained occultist, of course, has no such degree of control over his astral body and is more or less clumsy in his management of it. The Astral Body is always connected with the physical body (during the life of the latter) by a thin silk-like, astral thread, which maintains the communication between the two. Were this cord to be severed the physical body would die, as the connection of the soul with it would be terminated.

On this lower Astral Plane may also be perceived the auric colors of men, as described in our Fourth Lesson. Likewise it is on this plane that the emanations of thought may be observed by the clairvoyant vision, or the astral of one who visits that plane in his astral body. The mind is continually throwing off emanations, which extend some distance from the person, for a time, and which then, if strong enough, gradually pass off, drawn here and there by the corresponding thoughts of others. These thought emanations resemble clouds, some delicate and beautiful, while others are dark and murky. To the psychic or astral vision, places are seen to be filled with this thought-stuff, varying in character and appearance with the quality and nature of the original thought which produced them.

Some places are seen to be filled with bright attractive thought-stuff showing that the general character of the thought of those who inhabit it is of an uplifting and cheerful character, while other places are filled with a hazy, murky mass or cloud of thought-stuff, showing that those who live there (or some visitors) have been dwelling on the lower planes of thought, and have filled the place with depressing reminders of their sojourn there. Such rooms should be opened wide to the sun, and air, and one moving into them should endeavor to fill them with bright, cheerful and happy thoughts, which will drive out the lower quality of thought-stuff. A mental command, such as "I command you to move away from this place," will cause one to throw out strong thought vibrations, which will either dissolve the objectionable thought-stuff, or will cause it to be repelled and driven away from the immediate vicinity of the person making the command.

If people could see but for a few minutes the thought-atmosphere of groggeries, gambling-rooms, and places of that kind, they would not care to again visit them. Not only is the atmosphere fairly saturated with degrading thoughts, but the lower class of disembodied souls flock in large numbers around the congenial scene, striving to break the narrow bounds which separate them from the physical plane in such places.

Perhaps the best way to make plain to you the general aspects and phenomena of the Astral World,

would be to describe to you an imaginary trip made
by yourself in that world, in charge of an experienced occultist. We will send you, in imagination,
on such a trip, in this lesson, in charge of a competent guide—it being presupposed that you have
made considerable spiritual progress, as otherwise
even the guide could not take you very far, except
by adopting heroic and very unusual methods,
which he probably would not see fit to do in your
case. Are you ready for your trip? Well, here is
your guide.

You have gone into the silence, and suddenly become aware of having passed out of your body, and
to be now occupying only your astral body. You
stand beside your physical body, and see it sleeping
on the couch, but you realize you are connected
with it by a bright silvery thread, looking something like a large bit of bright spider-web. You are
conscious of the presence of your guide, who is to
conduct you on your journey. He also has left his
physical body, and is in his astral form, which re-
minds you of a vapory something, the shape of the
human body, but which can be seen through, and
which can move through solid objects at will. Your
guide takes your hand in his and says, "Come," and
in an instant you have left your room and are over
the city in which you dwell, floating along as does a
summer cloud. You begin to fear lest you may fall,
and as soon as the thought enters your mind you
find yourself sinking. But your guide places a hand
under you and sustains you, saying, "Now just real-

ize that you cannot sink unles you fear to—hold the thought that you are buoyant and you will be so." You do so, and are delighted to find that you may float at will, moving here and there in accordance to your wish or desire.

You see great volumes of thought-clouds arising from the city like great clouds of smoke, rolling along and settling here and there. You also see some finer vapory thought-clouds in certain quarters, which seem to have the property of scattering the dark clouds when they come in contact with them. Here and there you see bright thin lines of bright light, like an electric spark, traveling rapidly through space, which your guide tells you are telepathic messages passing from one person to another, the light being caused by the Prana with which the thought is charged. You see, as you descend toward the ground, that every person is surrounded by an egg-shaped body of color,—his aura—in which is reflected his thought and prevailing mental state, the character of the thought being represented by varying colors. Some are surrounded by beautiful auras, while others have around them a black, smoky aura, in which are seen flashes of red light. Some of these auras make you heart-sick to observe, as they give evidence of such base, gross, and animal thoughts, that they cause you pain, as you have become more sensitive now that you are out of your physical body. But you have not much time to spare here, as your trip is but a short one, and your guide bids you come on.

You do not seem to change your place in space, but a change seems to have come over everything— like the lifting of a gauzy curtain in the pantomime. You no longer see the physical world with its astral phenomena, but seem to be in a new world—a land of queer shapes. You see astral "shells" floating about—discarded astral bodies of those who have shed them as they passed on. These are not pleasant to look upon, and you hurry on with your guide, but before you leave this second ante-room to the real Astral World, your guide bids you relax your mental dependence upon your astral body, and much to your surprise you find yourself slipping out of it, leaving it in the world of shells, but being still connected with it by a silk-like cord, or thread, just as it, in turn, is connected with your physical body, which you have almost forgotten by this time, but to which you are still bound by these almost invisible ties. You pass on clothed in a new body, or rather an inner garment of ethereal matter, for it seems as if you have been merely shedding one cloak, and then another, the YOU part of yourself remains unchanged—you smile now at the recollection that once upon a time you thought that the body was "you." The plane of the "astral shells" fades away, and you seem to have entered a great room of sleeping forms, lying at rest and in peace, the only moving shapes being those from higher spheres who have descended to this plane in order to perform tasks for the good of their humbler brethren. Occasionally some sleeper will show

signs of awakening, and at once some of these helpers will cluster around him, and seem to melt away
into some other plane with him. But the most
wonderful thing about this region seems to be that
as the sleeper awakens slowly, his astral body slips
away from him just as did yours a little before, and
passes out of that plane to the place of "shells,"
where it slowly disintegrates and is resolved into its
original elements. This discarded shell is not connected with the physical body of the sleeping soul,
which physical body has been buried or cremated,
as it is "dead"; nor is the shell connected with the
soul which has gone on, as it has finally discarded it
and thrown it off. It is different in your case, for
you have merely left it in the ante-room, and will
return and resume its use, presently.

The scene again changes, and you find yourself in
the regions of the awakened souls, through which
you, with your guides, wander backward and forward. You notice that as the awakening souls pass
along, they seem to rapidly drop sheath after sheath
of their mental-bodies (for so these higher forms of
ethereal coverings are called) , and you notice that
as you move toward the higher planes your substance becomes more and more etherealized, and
that as you return to the lower planes it becomes
coarser and grosser, although always far more etherealized than even the astral body, and infinitely
finer than the material physical body. You also
notice that each awakening soul is left to finally
awaken on some particular plane. Your guide tells

you that the particular plane is determined by the
spiritual progress and attainment made by the soul
in its past lives (for it has had many earthly visits or
lives), and that it is practically impossible for a soul
to go beyond the plane to which it belongs, although
those on the upper planes may freely revisit the
lower planes, this being the rule of the Astral
World—not an arbitrary law, but a law of nature.
If the student will pardon the commonplace comparison, he may get an understanding of it, by imagining a large screen, or series of screens, such as
used for sorting coal into sizes. The large coal is
caught by the first screen, the next size by the sec
ond, and so on until the tiny coal is reached. Now
the large coal cannot get into the receptacle of the
smaller sizes, but the small sizes may easily pass
through the screen and join the large sizes, if force
be imparted to them. Just so in the Astral World,
the soul with the greatest amount of materiality,
and coarser nature, is stopped by the screen of a
certain plane, and cannot pass on the higher ones,
while one which has passed on to the higher planes,
having cast off more confining sheaths, can easily
pass backward and forward among the lower planes.
In fact souls often do so, for the purpose of visiting
friends on the lower planes, and giving them enjoy-
ment and comfort in this way, and, in cases of a
highly developed soul, much spiritual help may be
given in this way, by means of advice and instruction, when the soul on the lower plane is ready for
it. All of the planes, in fact, have Spiritual Help-

ers, from the very highest planes, some devoted souls preferring to so devote their time in the Astral World rather than to take a well earned rest, or to pursue certain studies for their own development. Your guide explains these things to you as you pass backward and forward, among the lower set of planes (the reason you do not go higher will be explained to you bye-and-bye), and he also informs you that the only exception to the rule of free passage to the planes below the plane of a soul, is the one which prevents the lower-plane souls from entering the "plane of the sleepers," which plane may not be entered by souls who have awakened on a low plane, but may be freely entered by those pure and exalted souls who have attained a high plane. The plane of the chamber of slumber is sacred to those occupying it, and those higher souls just mentioned, and is in fact in the nature of a distinct and separated state rather than one of the series of planes just mentioned.

The soul awakens on just the plane for which it is fitted—on just the sub-plane of that plane which its highest desires and tastes naturally select for it. It is surrounded by congenial minds, and is able to pursue that which the heart of the man had longed for during earth life. It may make considerable progress during this Astral World life, and so when it is reborn it is able to take a great step forward, when compared to its last incarnation. There are planes and sub-planes innumerable, and each finds an opportunity to develop and enjoy to the fullest the highest things of which it is capable at that particular period of development, and as we have said it may perfect itself and develop so that it will be born under much more favorable conditions and circumstances in the next earth life. But, alas, even in this higher world, all do not live up to their best, and instead of making the best of their opportunities, and growing spiritually, they allow their more material nature to draw them downward, and they spend much of their time on the planes beneath them, not to help and assist, but to live the less spiritual life of the denizens of the lower planes—the more material planes. In such cases the soul does not get the benefit of the Astral World sojourn and is born back into just about the same condition as the last earth-life—it is sent back to learn its lesson over again.

The very lowest planes of the Astral World are filled with souls of a gross type—undeveloped and animal like—who live as near as possible the lives they lived on earth (about the only thing they gain being the possibility of their "living-out" their gross tastes, and becoming sick and tired of it all, and thus allowing to develop a longing for higher things which will manifest in a "better-chance" when they are reborn). These undeveloped souls cannot, of course, visit the upper planes, and the only plane below them being the plane of shells and the astral sub-plane immediately above the material plane (which is one of the so-called anterooms of the Astral World) they often flock back as near to earth as is possible. They are able to get so near back to earth that they may become conscious of much that is transpiring there, particularly when the conditions are such that they are in harmony with their own natures. They may be said to be able to practically live on the low material plane, except that they are separated from it by a tantalizing thin veil, which prevents them from actively participating in it except on rare occasions. They may see, but not join in, the earth-life. They hang around the scenes of their old degrading lives, and often take possession of the brain of one of their own kind, who may be under the influence of liquor, and thus add to his own low desires. This is an unpleasant subject, and we do not care to dwell upon it—happily it does not concern those who read these lessons, as they have passed beyond this stage of development. Such low souls are so attracted by earth-life, on its lower planes, that their keen desires cause them to speedily reincarnate in similar conditions although there is always at least a slight improvement—there is never a going backward. A soul may make several attempts to advance, in spite of the dragging-back tendencies of its lower nature —but it never slips back quite as far as the place from which it started.

The souls in the higher planes, having far less attraction for earth-life, and having such excellent opportunities for advancement, naturally spend a much longer time in the Astral World, the general rule being that the higher the plane, the longer the rest and sojourn. But sooner or later the lesson is fully learned, and the soul yearns for that further advancement that can only come from the experience and action of another earth-life, and through the force of its desires (never against its will, remember) the soul is gradually caught in the current sweeping on toward rebirth, and becoming drowsy, is helped toward the plane of the room of slumber and, then falling into the soul-slumber it gradually "dies" to the Astral World, and is reborn into a new earth-life in accordance to its desires and tastes, and for which it is fit at that particular stage of its development. It does not fully awaken upon physical birth, but exists in a dreamy state of gradual awakening during the years of early childhood, its awakening being evidenced by the gradual dawning of intelligence in the child whose brain keeps pace with the demands made upon it. We will go more into detail regarding this matter, in the succeeding chapters.

All of these things, your guide has pointed out to you, and he has shown you examples of all the things we have just mentioned. You have met and talked with friends and loved ones who have passed out of the body and occupy some of the planes through which you have passed. You have noticed with wonder that these souls acted and spoke as if *their* life was the only natural one, and in fact seemed to think that you had come to them from some outside world. You also noticed that while those on each plane were more or less acquainted with the planes beneath them, they often seemed in total ignorance of those above them—except in the case of those on the higher planes who had awakened to a *conscious* realization of what it all meant, and knew that they were merely in a class working their way upward. Those on the lower planes seemed more or less unconscious of the real meaning of their existence, not having awakened to the conscious spiritual stage. You also noticed how few changes these souls seemed to have undergone— how very little more they seemed to know about things spiritual and occult than when on earth. You also noticed on the lower planes an old friend, who in earth-life, was a pronounced materialist, who did not seem to realize that he was "dead" and who believed that, by some catastrophe of nature, he had been transported to some other planet or physical world, and who was as keen as ever for his argument that "death ended all," and who flew into a rage with the visitors from the higher spheres who told him whom they were and from whence they came, calling them rogues and imposters, and demanding that they show him something of their claimed "higher spheres" if they were realities. He claimed that their sudden appearances and disappearances were simply the physical phenomena of the new planet upon which they were living. Passing away from him in the midst of his railing at you for agreeing with the "imposters" and "visionaries," who, to use his expression, were "little better than the spiritualists of the old world," you sadly asked your guide to take you to the highest spheres. Your guide smiled and said, "I will take you as far as you can go," and then took you to a plane which so fitted in with your desires, aspirations, tastes, and development, that you begged him to allow you to remain there, instead of taking you back to earth, as you felt that you had reached the "seventh heaven" of the Astral World. He insisted upon your return, but before starting told you that you were still in one of the sub-planes of the comparatively lower planes. You seemed to doubt his words, and like the materialist asked to be shown the greater things. He replied, "No, my son, you have progressed just as far as your limitations will allow—you have reached that part of the 'other life' which will be yours when you part with the body, unless you manage to develop still more and thus pass into a higher grade—thus far you may go but no farther. You have your limitations, just as I have mine, still farther on. No soul may travel beyond its spiritual boundaries."

"But," continued your guide, "beyond your plane and beyond mine are plane after plane, connected with our earth, the splendors of which man cannot conceive. And there are likewise many planes around the other planets of our chain—and there are millions of other worlds—and there are chains of universes just as there are chains of planets—and then greater groups of these chains—and so on greater and grander, beyond the power of man to imagine — on and on and on and on, higher and higher to inconceivable heights. An infinity of infinities of worlds are before us. Our world and our planetary chain and our system of suns, and our systems of solar systems, are but as grains of sand on the beach."

"Then what am I—poor mortal thing—lost among all this inconceivable greatness," you cried. "You are the most precious thing—a living soul," replied your guide, "and if you were destroyed the whole system of universes would crumble, for you are as necessary as the greatest part of it—it cannot do without you—you cannot be lost or destroyed— you are part of it all, and are eternal.

"And beyond all of this of which you have told me," you cried, "what is there, and what is the center of it all?" Your guide's face took on a rapt expression. "THE ABSOLUTE," he replied.

And when you reached your physical body again —just before your guide faded away—you asked him, "How many million miles away from Earth have we been, and how long were we gone?" He replied, "You never left the Earth at all—and your body was left alone but a moment of time—time and space belong not to the Astral world."

THE ELEVENTH LESSON.

BEYOND THE BORDER.

In these lessons we have not attempted to force upon the student any conception of the truth which did not appeal to him, or which did not harmonize with his own conception. We grant to all the liberty of their own convictions, preferring that they should accept only such of the Yogi teachings as may appeal to them, letting the rest pass by as not being needed just at that time. We merely state the Yogi's conception of the matter, as simply and plainly as we are able, that the student may understand the theory—whether or not it appeals to him as truth is a matter with which we have no concern. If it *is* true, then it *is* true, no matter what the student may think of it, and his belief or unbelief does not change matters. But, the Yogis do not hold to the idea that anyone is to be punished for unbelief, nor is one to be rewarded for belief—they hold that belief and unbelief are not matters of the will, but of the growth of understanding, therefore it is not consistent with Justice to suppose that one is rewarded or punished for belief or unbelief. The Yogis are the most tolerant of people. They see good, and truth, in all forms of belief, and conceptions of truth, and never blame any for not agreeing with them. They have no set creeds, and do not ask their followers to accept as a matter of course all that they teach. Their advice to students is: "Take what appeals to you, and leave the rest—tomorrow come back and take some of what you have rejected today, and so on, until you receive all we have to give you—do not force yourself to accept unpalatable truths, for when the time comes for you to receive them they will be pleasant to your mental taste —take what you please, and leave what you please —our idea of hospitality does not consist in forcing unpalatable things upon you, insisting that you must eat them to gain our favor, or that you will be punished for not liking them—take your own wherever you find it; but take nothing that is not yours by right of understanding; and fear not that anything that belongs to you may be withheld." With this understanding we proceed with our lesson —a most important one.

When the Ego leaves the body, at the moment of what we call Death, it leaves behind it the lower principles, and passes onward to states which will be considered by us presently. It leaves behind, first, the physical body. This physical body, as we have told you in the First Lesson, is composed of millions of tiny cells—little lives having a bit of mind or intelligence, under control of the central mind of the man; having also a supply of prana, or vital force, and a material casing or body, the sum of which little bodies makes the whole body of the man. We have devoted a chapter of our book upon "Hatha Yoga" to the consideration of these little lives, and we must refer the student to that book for fuller particulars of their life and work. When the death of the man occurs—when the Ego leaves its material sheath which it has used for the period of that particular "life," the cells separate and scatter, and that which we call decay sets in. The force which has held these cells together is withdrawn, and they are free to go their own way and form new combinations. Some are absorbed into the bodies of the plants in the vicinity, and eventually find themselves forming parts of the body of some animal which has eaten the plant, or a part of some other man who has eaten the plant or the meat of the animal which had eaten the plant. You will, of course, understand that these little cell-lives have nothing to do with the real soul or Ego of the man—they are but his late servants, and have no connection with his consciousness. Others of these atoms remain in the ground for some time, until taken up by some other form of living thing which needs nourishment. As a leading writer has said, "Death is but an aspect of life, and the destruction of one material form is but a prelude to the building up of another."

From the moment that the Ego leaves the physical body, and the influence of the commanding mind is withdrawn from the cells and the cellgroups, disorder reigns among them. They become a disorganized army, rushing hither and thither, interfering with each other—jostling and pushing each other—even fighting each other, their only object being to get away from the crowd—to escape from the general confusion. During the life of the body their main object is to work together in harmony, under the orders of their officers—after the death of the body their only object seems to separate and each go its own way. First the groups separate one from the other—then each group breaks up into smaller groups—and so on until each individual cell becomes freed from its fellows, and goes its own way, or where it is called by some form of life needing it. As a writer on the subject has said, "The body is never more alive when it is dead; but it is alive in its units, and dead in its totality."

When the Ego departs from the physical body, at the moment of death, the Prana being no longer under control of the central mind, responds only to the orders of the individual atoms or their groups, which have formed the individual body, and as the physical body disentegrates and is resolved into its original elements, each atom takes with it sufficient Prana to maintain its vitality, and to enable it to form new combinations, the unused Prana returning to the great universal storehouse, from which it came.

When the Ego leaves the body, at the moment of death, it carries with it the Astral Body as well as the higher principles. This astral body, you will remember, is the exact counterpart of the physical body, but is composed of a finer quality of matter, and is invisible to the ordinary vision, but may be plainly seen by clairvoyant or astral sight, and may therefore be sometimes seen by persons under certain psychic conditions. Clairvoyants describe the parting of the Astral Body from the Physical Body as most interesting. They describe it as rising from the physical body, like a cloud of thin luminous vapor, but being connected with the physical body by a slender, silken, vapory cord, which cord becomes thinner and thinner until it becomes invisible to even the fine clairvoyant vision, just before it breaks entirely. The Astral Body exists some time after the physical death of the man, and under certain circumstances it becomes visible to living persons, and is called a "ghost." The Astral Body of a dying person is sometimes projected by an earnest desire and may become visible to relatives or friends with whom the dead man is in sympathy.

After a time, differing in various cases, as we will see later on, the Astral Body is discarded by the Ego, and it in turn begins to disintegrate. This discarded Astral Body is nothing more than a corpse of finer material, and is what occultists know as an "astral shell." It has no life or intelligence, when thus discarded, and floats around in the lower astral atmosphere, until it is resolved into its original elements. It seems to have a peculiar attraction toward its late physical counterpart, and will often return to the neighborhood of the physical body and disintegrate with it. Persons of psychic sight, either normal or influenced by fear or similar

emotions, frequently see these astral shells floating
around graveyards, over battlefields, etc., and are
often mistaken for the "spirits" of departed people,
whereas they are no more the person than is the
physical corpse beneath the ground. These astral
shells may be "galvanized" into a semblance of life
by coming into contact with the vitality of some
"medium," the prana of the latter animating it,
and the sub-conscious mentality of the medium
causing it to manifest signs of life and partial intelligence. At some of the seances of the mediums
these astral shells are materialized by means of the
vitality of the medium, and talk in a stupid, discon-
nected way with those around, but it is not the
person himself talking, but a mere shell animated
by the life principle of the medium and the "circle," and acting and talking like an automaton.
There are, of course, other forms of spirit return,
which are far different, but those investigating
spiritualistic phenomena should beware of con-
founding these astral shells with the real intelligence of their deceased friends. And now let us return to the Ego, which has left the physical body.

While the Ego, encased in its Astral body, is
slowly passing out of the Physical Body, the whole
life of the person from infancy to old age, passes before his mental vision. The memory gives up its
secrets, and picture after picture passes in swift succession before the mind, and many things are made
plain to the departing soul—the reason of many
things is discovered, and the soul sees what it all

means—that is, it understands its whole life just complete, because it sees it as a whole. This is in the nature of a vivid dream to the dying individual, but it leaves a deep impress, and the memories are recalled and made use of at a later period, by the soul. Occultists have always urged that the friends and relatives of a dying person should maintain quiet and calm around him, that he may not be disturbed by conflicting emotions, or distracting sounds. The soul should be allowed to go on its way in peace and quiet, without being held back by the wishes or conversation of those around him.

So the Ego passes on, and out from the body. To where? Let us say here that the future states of the soul, between incarnations, have nothing to do with places—it is a matter of "states" not of places. There are numerous places of existence, and all interpenetrate each other, so that a given space may contain intelligences living on several different planes, those living on the lower planes not being conscious of the existence and presence of those living on the higher ones. So get the idea of "place" out of your minds—it is all a matter of "states," or "planes."

The soul after passing out of the body, if left undisturbed by emphatic calls from those whom it has left behind (and which calls may consist of violent manifestations of grief, and earnest demands for the return of the departed one on the part of some loved one, or from someone to whom the deceased person was bound by ties of duty) falls into a semi-conscious state—a blissful, peaceful, happy, restful state—a dream of the soul. This state continues for some time (varying in individuals as we shall see) until the astral shell falls from it, and floats off in the astral atmosphere, and until the lower portions of that etherealized-matter which confines the lower portions of the mind gradually dissolves and also drops from the soul, leaving it possessed of only the higher portions of its mentality.

The man of low spiritual development, and consequently of a larger degree of animal nature, will part with but little of his mind-body, and soon reaches the highest of which he has been mentally and spiritually capable in his earth-life. The man of high spiritual attainment, will gradually "shed" much of his mental-body, until he has thrown off all except the highest portions developed in his earth life. Those between the two mentioned types will act according to their degree of spiritual attainment, of course. Then, when the last possible remnant of the lower mentality has dropped from the soul, it awakes, as it passes on to states which will be described a little later on in this lesson. It will be seen that the man of gross mentality and spiritual development will stay in the dream-like state but a short time, as the process of casting off of sheaths is a comparatively simple one, requiring but little time. And it likewise will be seen that the man who has reached a high degree of spiritual development, will rest for a longer period, as he has much more to get rid of, and this discarded material of the mind drops from him like the leaves of a rose, one after the other, from the outer to the inner. Each soul awakens when it has discarded all that it can (or rather all that *will* drop from it) and when it has reached the highest state possible to it. Those who have made material spiritual progress during the earth-life just past, will have much useless and outgrown matter to discard, while the one who has neglected his opportunities, and dies about as he was born, will have but little to throw off, and will awaken in a very short time. Each rests until the highest point of unfoldment has manifested itself. But before going on further, let us stop a moment to say that both the sinking into the restful state, and the soundness and continuance of it may be interfered with by those left in the earth life. A soul which has "something on its mind" to communicate, or which is grieved by the pain of those who have been left behind (especially if it hears the lamentations and constant call for its return) will fight off the dreamy state creeping over it, and will make desperate efforts to return. And, likewise, the mental calls of those who have been left behind, will disturb the slumber, when it has been once entered into, and will cause the sleeping soul to rouse itself and endeavor to answer the calls, or at least will partially awaken it and retard its unfoldment. These half-awake souls often manifest in spiritualistic circles. Our selfish grief and demands often cause our loved ones who have passed

much pain and sorrow and unrest, unless they have
learned the true state of affairs before they have
passed out, and refuse to be called back to earth
even by those they love. Cases are known to occultists where souls have fought off the slumber for
years in order to be around their loved ones on
earth, but this course was unwise as it caused unnecessary sorrow and pain to both the one who
had passed on, and those who had remained on
earth. We should avoid delaying the process of
those who have passed on—let them sleep on and
rest, awaiting the hour of their transformation. It is
like making them die their death several times in
succession—those who truly love and understand
avoid this—their love and understanding bids them
let the soul depart in peace and take its well earned
rest and gain its full development. This period of
soul-slumber is like the existence of the babe in its
mother's womb—it sleeps that it may awaken into
life and strength.

Before passing on to the awakening, however, we
think it proper to state that it is only the soul of the
person who has died a natural death which sinks at
once (if not disturbed) into the soul-slumber.
Those who die by "accident," or who are killed—in
other words, those who pass out of the body suddenly, find themselves wide-awake and in full possession of the mental faculties for some time. They
often are not aware that they have "died," and
cannot understand what is the matter with them.
They are often fully conscious (for a short time)

of life on earth, and can see and hear all that is going on around them, by means of their astral faculties. They cannot imagine that they have passed out of the body, and are sorely perplexed. Their lot would be most unhappy for a few days, until the sleep overtook them were it not for the Astral Helpers, who are souls from the higher states of existence, who gather around them and gently break to them the news of their real condition—offer them words of comfort and advice, and "take care" of them until they sink into the soul-slumber just as a tired child sinks to sleep at night. These helpers never fail in their duty, and no one who passes out suddenly is neglected, be he or she "good" or "bad," for these Helpers know that all are God's children and their own brothers and sisters. Men of high spiritual development and powers have been known to pass out of their physical bodies temporarily (by means of their Astral Bodies) for the purpose of giving aid and advice in times of great catastrophes, or after a great battle, when immediate assistance and advice are needed. At such times, also, some of the higher intelligences in the scale of spiritual evolution descend from their lofty states and appearing as men give words of encouragement and the benefit of their wisdom. This not only in civilized countries but in all parts of the world, for all are akin. Many who have reached the high stages of spiritual development, and who have advanced far beyond the rest of the particular race-group to which they belong, and who have earned a longer stay in the higher states, awaiting the progress of their brothers, devote themselves to this and similar tasks, voluntarily relinquishing their earned rest and happiness for the good of their less fortunate brethren. Persons dying in the way of which we have spoken, of course, gradually fall into the slumber of the soul, and the process of the casting off of the confining sheaths goes on just as in cases of those dying a "natural" death.

When the soul has cast off the confining sheaths, and has reached the state for which it is prepared by its earth-lives, including that gained by development in the last earth-life, it passes immediately to the plane in the Astral World for which it is fitted, and to which it is drawn by the Law of Attraction. Now the Astral World, in all of its stages and planes, is not a "place" but a state, as we have before stated. These planes interpenetrate and those dwelling on one plane are not conscious of those dwelling on another, nor can they pass from one plane to another, with this exception—those dwelling on a higher plane are able to see (if they desire) the planes below them in the order of development, and may also visit the lower planes, if they desire to do so. But those on the lower planes are not able to either see or visit the higher planes. This is not because there is a "watchman at the gate," or anything of that sort (for there can be no "gate" to a plane or state) but from the same reason that a fish is not able to soar above the water

into the air like a bird—its nature does not permit
it to do so. A soul having another soul toward
which it is attached by some old tie, and finding
that soul on a lower plane than itself, is able to
visit the less developed soul and aid it in its development by advice and instruction, and to thus prepare it for its next incarnation so that when the two
shall meet again in earth-life the less developed
soul will have grown far nearer to its higher
brother- or sister-soul, and may thereafter go hand
in hand throughout life, or lives. This, of course,
providing the less developed soul is willing to be
instructed. Souls after reaching a certain degree of
development are quite willing to be instructed
when out of the body (as above stated) as they are
freed from the distracting influences of earth-life,
and are more open to the help of the Spirit. The
Yogi teaching goes so far as to state that in rare
cases, the helping soul may even bring his lower
brother to such a state that he is enabled to throw
off some of the lower mental principles which have
clung to him after his awakening, and which kept
him in a certain plane, and thus enable him to pass
on to the next higher plane. But this is rare, and
can only happen when the soul has been *nearly* but
not quite able to throw off the confining sheath,
unaided.

The lower planes of the Astral World are filled
with souls of a gross, undeveloped type, who live
lives very similar to those lived on earth. In fact
they are so closely connected with the material

plane, and are so attracted to it, that they are so conscious of much that goes on in it, that they may be said to be living on the material plane, and only prevented from active participation in it by a thin veil which separates them from their own kind in the body. These souls hang around the old scenes of their earthly degradation, and often influence one of their kind who is under the influence of liquor and who is thereby open to influences of this nature. They live their old lives over again in this way, and add to the brutality and degradation of the living by their influences and association. There are quite a number of these lower planes, as well as the higher planes, each containing disembodied souls of the particular class belonging to it. These lower plane souls are in very close contact with the material plane, and are consequently the ones often attracted to seances, where the medium and sitters are on a low plane. They masquerade as the "spirits" of friends of visitors, and others, often claiming to be some well known and celebrated personages. They play the silly pranks so often seen at seances, and take a particular delight in such things, and "general devilment," if permitted to do so. They are not fit company for people on the higher plane, whether they be embodied or disembodied.

These lower plane souls spend but little time in the disembodied state, and are strongly attracted by the material life, the consequence being that they are filled with a great desire to reincarnate,

and generally spend but little time between two incarnations. Of course, when they are reborn they
are attracted to, and attracted by, parents of the
same tendencies, so that the surroundings in their
new earth-life will correspond very closely to those
of their old one. These crude and undeveloped
souls, as well as the souls of the savage races, progress but slowly, making but a trifling advance in
each life, and having to undergo repeated and frequent incarnations in order to make even a little
progress. Their desires are strong for the material,
and they are attracted to and by it—the Spirit's
influences exerting but a comparatively slight
attraction upon them. But even these make *some*
progress—all are moving forward if even but a
little.

The souls on each of the succeeding higher
planes, of course, make more rapid progress each
earth-life, and have fewer incarnations, and a much
longer time between them. Their inclinations and
tastes being of a higher order, they prefer to dwell
on in the higher places of disembodied life, thinking of and contemplating the higher teachings,
aided as they are by the absence from material
things and encouraged by the rays of the Spiritual
Mind beating down upon them, helping their unfoldment. They are able to prepare themselves for
great progress in this way, and often spend centuries on the higher planes, before reincarnating. In
some cases where they have advanced far beyond
their race, they spend thousands of years in the

higher planes, waiting until the race grows up to render their rebirth attractive, and in the meantime they find much helpful work to do for less developed souls.

But sooner or later, the souls feel a desire to gain new experiences, and to manifest in earth-life some of the advancement which has come to them since "death," and for these reasons, and from the attraction of desires which have been smoldering there, not lived out or cast off, or, possibly influenced by the fact that some loved soul, on a lower plane, is ready to incarnate and wishing to be incarnated at the same time in order to be with it (which is also a desire) the souls fall into the current sweeping toward rebirth, and the selection of proper parents and advantageous circumstances and surroundings, and in consequence again fall into a soul-slumber, gradually, and so when their time comes they "die" to the plane upon which they have been existing and are "born" into a new physical life and body. A soul does not fully awaken from its sleep immediately at birth, but exists in a dream-like state during the days of infancy, its gradual awakening being evidenced by the growing intelligence of the babe, the brain of the child keeping pace with the demands made upon it. In some case the awakening is premature, and we see cases of prodigies, child-genius, etc., but such cases are more or less abnormal, and unhealthy. Occasionally the dreaming soul in the child half-awakes, and startles us by some profound observation, or mature remark or conduct.

Much of this process of preparing for reincarnation is performed by the soul unconsciously, in obedience to its inspirations, and desires, as it really has not grown to understand what it all means, and what is before it, and is being swept along by the Law of Attraction almost unconsciously. But after souls attain a certain degree of development, they become conscious of the process of reincarnation, and are thereafter conscious of past lives, and preceding a rebirth may take a conscious part in selecting the environments and surroundings. The higher they rise in the scale, the greater their conscious power, and choice.

It will readily be seen that there are planes upon planes of disembodied existence. The Yogi Philosophy teaches that there are Seven Great Planes (sometimes spoken of by uneducated Hindus as the "seven heavens"), but each great plane has seven sub-divisions, and each sub-division has seven minor divisions, and so on.

It is impossible for us to begin to describe the nature of the higher astral life. We have no words to describe it, and no minds to comprehend it. Life on the lower planes is very similar to earth-life, many of the inhabitants seeming to think that it is a part of the earth, and, not realizing that they are freed from earthly limitations, imagine that fire can burn them, water can drown them, etc. They live practically on the earth amidst its scenes. Above these are planes whose inhabitants have higher ideas and lives—and so on and on and on, until the bliss of the higher planes cannot be comprehended by man today. In some of the intermediate planes, those who are fond of music indulge to the utmost their love for it—artists their love for their art— intellectual workers pursue their studies—and so on, along these lines. Above these are those who have awakened spiritually and have opportunities for developing themselves, and gaining knowledge. Above these are states of which we cannot dream. And, yet remember this, even these highest planes are but parts of the high Astral Plane, which plane is but one of the lower ones of the Universe, and above that comes plane after plane of existence. But why speak of this, friends—we cannot undertake to master the problem of higher mathematics, when we scarcely know how to add two figures together. But all this is for us—all for us—and we cannot be robbed of our inheritance.

THE TWELFTH LESSON.

SPIRITUAL EVOLUTION.

The beautiful doctrine of Spiritual Evolution—
that gem in the diadem of the Yogi Philosophy—
is sadly misunderstood and misinterpreted, even
by many who are its friends. The mass of unin-
formed people confuse it with the crudest ideas of
the ignorant races of Asia and Africa—believe that
it teaches that the souls of men descend into the
bodies of the lower animals after death. And under
the guise of high teachings regarding Reincarnation, many promulgate theories holding that the
soul of man is bound to the wheel of human rebirth, and must live in body after body—whether
it will or not—until certain great cycles are past,
when the race moves on to another planet. All of
these misconceptions, however, are based upon the
real truth—they are the truth, but not the *whole*
truth. It is true that the soul of a brutal, selfish, bestial man, after death, will be drawn *by the force of
its own desires* toward rebirth in the body of some
of the lower and more beast-like races of man—it
has failed in its class-work, and has been sent back
to a lower grade. But the soul that has once reached
the stage of even primitive Manhood, never can

sink back into the plane of lower animal-life. As bestial as it may be, it still has acquired something that the animal lacks, and that something it can never lose. And likewise, although the race—as a race—must wait until certain periods are reached before it may move onward, yet the individual who has risen beyond the need of immediate rebirth, is not compelled to reincarnate as a man of the present stage of development, but may wait until the race "catches up" to him, as it were, when he may join it in its upward swing, the intervening period being spent either in the higher planes of the Astral World or in *conscious* temporary so journ in other material spheres, helping in the great work of the evolution of all Life.

And, so far from the spiritually awakened Man being compelled to suffer continuous involuntary rebirths, he is not reborn except with his own consent and desire, and with a continuance of consciousness—this continuance of consciousness depending upon the spiritual attainment reached. Many who read these lines are partially conscious of their past existences in the flesh, and their attraction to this subject is due to that semi-consciousness and recognition of the truth. Others, now in the flesh, have varying degrees of consciousness, reaching, in some cases, a full recollection of their past lives. And, rest assured, dear student, that when you reach a certain stage of spiritual awakening (and you may have reached it even now) you will have left behind you unconscious rebirth, and, after you have passed out of your present body—and after a period of spiritual rest—you will not be reborn, until you are ready and willing, and you will then carry with you a continuous recollection of all that you choose to carry with you into your new life. So cease this fretting about forced rebirth, and stop worrying about your fancied loss of consciousness in future lives. Spiritual attainment is slow and arduous, but every inch gained is so much further on, and you can never slip back, nor lose the slightest part of what you've gained.

Even those who are reborn, unconsciously, as are the majority of the race, are not actually reborn against their will or desire. On the contrary, they are reborn *because* they desire it—because their tastes and desires create longings that only renewed life in the flesh can satisfy, and, although they are not fully conscious of it, they place themselves again within the operation of the Law of Attraction, and are swept on to a rebirth, in just the surroundings best calculated to enable them to exhaust their desires, and satisfy their longings—these desires and longings thus dying a natural death, and making way for higher ones. So long as people earnestly desire material things—the things of the flesh and the material life, and are not able to divorce themselves from such things at will—just so long will they be drawn toward rebirth that these desires may be gratified or satisfied. But when one has,

by experience in many lives, learned to see things
as they are, and to recognize that such things are
not a part of his real nature, then the earnest
desire grows less and finally dies, and that person
escapes from the operation of the Law of Attraction, and need not undergo rebirth until some
higher desire or aspiration is appealed to, as the
evolution of the race brings new eras and peoples.
It is as if one were to soar away up above the atmosphere of the earth—beyond the sphere of the earth's
attraction—and would then wait until the earth re-
volved beneath him and he saw, far below, the spot
which he wished to visit, when all he would have to
do would be to allow himself to sink until the force
of gravity exerted by the earth would draw him to
the desired place.

The idea of compulsory rebirth is horrible to the
mind of the average man, and rightly so, for it
violates his intuitive sense of the justice and truth
of this great law of Life. We are here because we
wished to be—in obedience to the Law of Attraction, operating in accordance with our desires and
aspiration—yes, often, longings—after our departure
from our last fleshly tenement, and the period of
rest which always follows a life. And we will never
be anywhere else, or in any other life, unless by
reason of that same law, called into effect in the
same manner. It is quite true, that the period
between lives gives us an opportunity to receive the
higher knowledge of the Spirit more clearly than
when disturbed by material things, but even with

this additional aid, our desires are often sufficiently strong to cause us to reject the gentle promptings of the Spirit, as to what is best for us (just as we do in our everyday lives) and we allow ourselves to be caught up in the current of desire, and are swept onward toward rebirth in such conditions as to allow us to manifest and express those desires and longings. Sometimes, the Spirit's voice influences us to a degree, and we are born in conditions representing a compromise between the Spirit's teaching and the grosser desires, and the result is often a life torn with conflicting desires and restless longings—but all this is a promise of better conditions in the future.

When one has developed so far as to be open to the influence of the Spiritual Mind in his physical life, he may rest assured that his next choice of rebirth will be made with the full approval and wisdom of that higher part of his mind, and the old mistakes will be obviated.

As a general statement of truth, we may say that those who actually *feel* within them that consciousness of having always existed and of being intended for an endless existence, need fear nothing on the score of future unconscious rebirths. They have reached the stage of consciousness in which, henceforth, they will be aware of the whole process of the future incarnations, and will make the change (if they wish to) just as one changes his place of residence, or travels from one country to another. They are "delivered" from the necessity of the unconscious rebirth, from blind desire, which has been their portion in the past, and which is the lot of the majority of the race.

And now after this long preamble, let us see what Spiritual Evolution, as taught by the Yogis, really means.

The Yogi Philosophy teaches that Man has always lived and always will live. That that which we call Death is but a falling to sleep to awaken the following morning. That Death is but a temporary loss of consciousness. That life is continuous, and that its object is development, growth, unfoldment. That we are in Eternity Now as much as we ever can be. That the Soul is the Real Man, and not merely an appendage or attachment to his physical body, as many seem to regard it. That the Soul may exist equally well out of the body as in it, although certain experience and knowledge may be obtained only by reason of a physical existence—hence that existence. That we have bodies now, just because we need them—when we have progressed beyond a certain point, we will not need the kind of bodies we have now, and will be relieved of them. That on the grosser planes of life far more material bodies than ours were occupied by the soul—that on higher planes the soul will occupy finer bodies. That as we live out the experiences of one earth life, we pass out of the body into a state of rest, and after that are reborn into bodies, and into conditions, in accordance with our needs and desires. That the real Life is really a succession of lives—of rebirths, and that our present life is merely one of a countless number of previous lives, our present self being the result of the experiences gained in our previous existences.

The Yogi Philosophy teaches that the Soul has existed for ages, working its way up through innumerable forms, from lower to higher,—always progressing, always unfolding. That it will continue to develop and unfold, through countless ages, in many forms and phases, but always higher and higher. The Universe is great and large, and there are countless worlds and spheres for its inhabitants, and we shall not be bound to earth one moment after we are fitted to move on to higher spheres and planes. The Yogis teach that while the majority of the race are in the unconscious stage of Spiritual Evolution, still there are many awakening to the truth, and developing a spiritual consciousness of the real nature and future of Man, and that these spiritually awakened people will never again have to go through the chain of continued unconscious rebirth, but that their future development will be on a conscious plane, and that they will enjoy to the full the constant progression and development, instead of being mere pawns on the chessboard of Life. The Yogis teach that there are many forms of life, much lower than Man—so much lower that we cannot conceive of them. And that there are degrees of life so far above our present plane of development that our minds cannot grasp the idea. Those souls who have traveled over the

Path which we are now treading—our Elder Brothers—are constantly giving us their aid and encouragement, and are often extending to us the helping hand—although we recognize it not. There are in existence, on planes beyond our own, intelligences which were once men as are we, but who have now progressed so far in the scale that compared with us they are angels and archangels—and we shall be like unto them sometime.

The Yogi Philosophy teaches that YOU who are reading these lines, have lived many, many lives. You have lived in the lower forms of life, working your way up gradually in the scale. After you passed into the human phase of existence you lived as the caveman, the cliff dweller, the savage, the barbarian; the warrior, the knight; the priest; the scholar of the Middle Ages;—now in Europe; now in India; now in Persia; now in the East; now in the West. In all ages,—in all climes—among all peoples —of all races—have you lived, had your existence, played your part, and died. In each life have you gained experiences; learned your lessons; profited by your mistakes; grown, developed and unfolded. And when you passed out of the body, and entered into the period of rest between incarnations, your memory of the past life gradually faded away, but left in its place the result of the experiences you had gained in it. Just as you may not remember much about a certain day, or week, twenty years ago, still the experiences of that day or week have left indelible traces upon your character, and have influenced your every action since—so while you may have forgotten the details of your previous existences, still have they left their impress upon your soul, and your everyday life now is just what it is by reason of those past experiences.

After each life there is sort of a boiling down of the experiences, and the result—the real result of the experience—goes to make up a part of the new self—the improved self—which will after a while seek a new body into which to reincarnate. But with many of us there is not a total loss of memory of past lives—as we progress we bring with us a little more of consciousness each time—and many of us to-day have occasional glimpses of remembrance of some past existence. We see a scene for the first time, and it seems wonderfully familiar, and yet we cannot have seen it before. There is sort of a haunting memory which disturbs. We may see a painting—some old masterpiece—and we feel instinctively as if we had gazed upon it away in the dim past, and yet we have never been near it before. We read some old book, and it seems like an old friend, and yet we have no recollection of ever having seen it in our present life. We hear some philosophical theory, and we immediately "take to it," as if it were something known and loved in our childhood. Some of us learn certain things as if we were relearning them—and indeed such is the case. Children are born and develop into great musicians, artists, writers or artisans, from early childhood, even though their parents possessed no talents of the kind. Shakespeares spring from the families whose members possess no talents, and astonish the world. Abraham Lincolns come from similar walks of life, and when responsibility is placed upon them show the greatest genius. These and many similar things can be explained only upon the theory of previous existence. We meet people for the first time, and the conviction is borne upon us, irresistibly, in spite of our protests, that we have known them before—that they have been something to us in the past, but when, oh! when?

Certain studies come quite easy to us, while others have to be mastered by hard labor. Certain occupations seem the most congenial to us, and no matter how many obstacles are placed in the way, we still work our way to the congenial work. We are confronted with some unforeseen obstacle, or circumstances call for the display of unusual power or qualities on our part, and lo! we find that we have the ability to perform the task. Some of the greatest writers and orators have discovered their talents "by accident." All of these things are explained by the theory of Spiritual Evolution. If heredity is everything, how does it happen that several children of the same parents differ so widely from each other, from their parents, and from the relations on both sides of the house? Is it all heredity or reversion? Then pray tell us from whom did Shakespeare inherit—to whom did he revert?

Argument after argument might be piled up to

prove the reasonableness of rebirth, but what would it avail? Man might grasp it intellectually and admit that it was a reasonable working hypothesis, but what intellectual conception ever gave peace to the soul—gave it that sense of reality and truth that would enable it to go down in the valley of the shadow of death without faltering—with a smile on its face? No! such certainty comes only from the light which the Spiritual Mind sheds upon the lower mental faculties. The intellect may arrange the facts, and deduce a course of action from them, but the soul is satisfied only with the teachings of the Spirit, and until it receives them must feel that unrest and uncertainty that comes when the intellect unfolds and asks that mighty question "Why?" which it by itself cannot answer.

The only answer to the query "Is re-birth a fact," is "Does your soul recognize it as such?" Until the soul feels of itself that the theory is true—because it coincides with that inner conviction, there is no use in arguing the matter. The soul must recognize it for itself—must answer its own question. It is true that the presentation of the theory (we call it a "theory" although the Yogis know it is a *fact*) will awaken memories in the mind of some—may give them the courage to consider as reasonable the half-formed thoughts and queries which had floated around in their minds for years—but that is all it can do. Until the soul grasps and "feels" the truth of rebirth, it must wander around working on the subconscious plane of life, having rebirth forced upon it by its own desires and longings, losing consciousness to a great extent. But after the soul has begun to "feel" the truth, it is never the same— it carries with it memories of the past, sometimes faint and sometimes clear—and it begins to manifest a *conscious* choice in the matter of rebirth. Just as does the plant work on the sub-conscious plane, and the animal on a semi-conscious plane— and the man on the gradually increasing planes of consciousness, so does man gradually evolve from the sub-conscious stage of rebirth, on to the semi-conscious plane, and then on and on, increasing his consciousness from time to time, until he lives on the conscious plane, both in his physical life, and during the rest period, and in the new birth. There are men among us to-day (few, it is true, but many more than most people imagine) who are fully conscious of the past existences, and who have been so since early childhood, only that their days of infancy were passed in a dreamlike state, until their physical brains were sufficiently developed to enable the soul to think clearly. In fact, many children seem to have a dim consciousness of the past, but fearing the comments of their elders, learn to stifle these bits of remembrance until they fail to evoke them.

Those who have not awakened to the truth of rebirth, cannot have it forced upon them by argument, and those who "feel" the truth of it do not need the argument. So we have not attempted to argue the matter in this short presentation of the theory. Those who are reading this lesson are attracted toward the subject by reason of interest awakened in some past life, and they really feel that there must be some truth in it, although they may not as yet have arrived at a point where they can fully assimilate it.

Many of those upon whom the truth of the proposition is borne home by their inmost feelings or fragmentary recollections evince a disinclination to fully accept it. They fear the idea of being reborn without their consent or knowledge. But as we have stated to them, this is a groundless fear, for, if they are really beginning to "feel" the truth of rebirth, their period of sub-conscious manifestation on that plane is passing away.

Many say that they have no desire to live again, but they really mean that they would not like to live just the same life that they have—of course not, they do not want the same experiences over again —but if there is a single thing in life that they would like; a single position they would like to fill; a single desire that they feel needs to be satisfied in order to make them happy,—then they do really want to live again to secure the missing thing. They are here because they wanted to be here—or had desires which cried for satisfaction—and they will live again in just the circumstances needed to gratify their desires or wishes, or that are likely to give them the necessary experience for higher spiritual growth.

To the student of this subject of Spiritual Evolution, a great world of interesting facts open itself. Light is thrown upon history and the progress of mankind, and a most fascinating field of research is presented. We must resist the temptation to go into this branch of the subject, as it would lead us in attractive paths which we are forbidden to take up in these elementary lessons owing to the lack of space. We may find room, however, to say a little about these matters.

The earth is one of a chain of planets, belonging to our solar system, all of which are intimately connected with the others in this great law of Spiritual Evolution. Great waves of life sweep over the chain, carrying race after race along the chain, from one planet to another. Each race stays on each planet for a certain period, and then having developed, passes on to the planet next highest in the scale of evolution, finding there conditions best suited for its development. But this progress from planet to planet is not circular—it resembles a spiral, circling round and round and yet rising higher with each curve.

Let us suppose a soul dwelling upon any of the planets of our planetary chain, in a comparatively undeveloped state of spiritual growth—occupying a low place in the scale of evolution. The soul gains the experiences coming to it in that stage, in a number of incarnations, and then is swept away toward the next highest planet in the chain, together with the rest of its particular race, and is reincarnated there. In this new home it occupies a plane distinctly in advance of the one occupied in the last one—its entire race forming the nucleus of a new race there, some being pioneers while the others follow after. But still this advanced stage (as compared with its stage on the planet just left behind it) may be much lower in the scale of progress than other races dwelling on the same planet with it. Some of the races, lowest in the point of evolution on this earth, may have been much nearer the highest stage of development on the last planet inhabited by them, and still they have progressed greatly by the change—the highest on a lower planet perhaps being less highly developed than the lowest on one farther along the planetary chain. Many of the races that formerly inhabited the Earth, traces of whom we occasionally find, have passed on to a higher stage of development. History shows us that race after race came to the front in the earth's development—played their part upon the stage of action—and then passed on—where? The occult philosophies furnish the missing link of explanation. And our race has grown from the stone-age stage—and still further back—and will continue to progress—and will then pass on, making way for some newer race which may be even now sending out pioneers from some other planet.

This does not mean, necessarily, that each race that history tells us of has passed from the earth. On the contrary, occultists know that some, and in fact most of the races known to history, have incarnated in some of the races today. The confusion is explained by the fact that each race has several sub-races, which really belong to the main race. For instance, occultists know that the ancient Egyptians—the Romans—the Greeks—the Atlanteans—the ancient Persians, etc., etc., are now living on this earth—that is the souls which formerly incarnated in these races, are now incarnated in some of the modern races. But there are other races—prehistoric races—which have passed away from the earth's attraction entirely, and have gone on to the higher planes of action in the higher planets. There are a number of planets lower in the scale of progress than our earth, and there are several higher, toward which we are moving. There are of course, other solar systems—other chains of suns—other sub-Universes (if we may be pardoned for using the term), and all this is ahead of every soul, no matter how lowly or how humble.

Our race, at present, is going through a most important period of evolution. It is passing from the unconscious stage of spiritual development, into the conscious stage. Many have already attained their conscious stage, and many more are awakening to it. The whole race will ultimately have it, this being precedent to their moving on. This gradual awakening to spiritual consciousness, is what is causing all this unrest in the world of thought— this breaking away from old ideals and forms—this hunger for the truth—this running to and fro after new truths, and old truths restated. It is a critical period in the history of the race, and many hold that it implies a possible division of the race into two sub-races, one of whom will be possessed of spiritual consciousness, and will move on ahead of the remaining sub-race of slower brothers, who must work up by degrees. But the race will again be united, before it finally passes on from the earth, as it is bound together by the Law of Spiritual Cause and Effect. We are all interested in each other's progress—not only because we are brothers but because our own soul must wait until the whole race develops. Of course the more rapidly developed soul does not have to be reincarnated simply because its slower brother has to do so. On the contrary the highly developed soul spends a long period of waiting on the higher planes of the Astral World while its slower brother works out his evolution in repeated births, the sojourn in the higher planes giving the developed soul great happiness and benefit, as explained in other lessons. Many of these "waiting souls," however, choose to sacrifice their well-earned rest, by coming back to earth to help and uplift their brethren, either in the form of Astral Helpers, or even by a deliberate and conscious re-birth (which is not needed for their development) they deliberately taking on the body of flesh, with all its burdens, in order to assist their weaker brothers toward the goal. The great teachers of the races, have been largely composed of these self-sacrificing souls, who voluntarily "renounced heaven" for the love of their fellow man. It is very hard to imagine what a great sacrifice this is—this coming back to a comparatively low developed civilization, from a high plane of spiritual development. It is like Emerson doing missionary work among the Bushmen.

Toward what goal is all this evolution tending? What does it all mean? From the low forms of life, to the highest—all are on The Path. To what place or state does The Path lead? Let us attempt to answer by asking you to imagine a series of millions of circles one within the other. Each circle means a stage of life. The outer circles are filled with life in its lowest and most material stages—each circle nearer the center holding higher and higher forms—until men (or what were men) become as gods. Still on, and on, does the form of life grow higher, until the human mind cannot grasp the idea. And what is in the center? The brain of the entire Spiritual Body—The Absolute —God!

And we are traveling toward that center!

THE THIRTEENTH LESSON.

SPIRITUAL CAUSE AND EFFECT.

Life is the constant accumulation of knowledge—
the storing up of the result of experiences. The
law of cause and effect is in constant operation, and
we reap what we sow—not as a matter of punishment, but as the effect following the cause. The-
ology teaches us that we are punished *for* our sins,
but the higher knowledge shows us that we are
punished *by* our mistakes instead of *for* them. The
child who touches the hot stove is punished by
reason of the act itself, not by some higher power
for having "sinned." Sin is largely a matter of ignorance and mistake. Those who have reached the
higher plane of spiritual knowledge have borne
upon them such a convincing knowledge of the
folly and unwisdom of certain acts and thoughts,
that it becomes almost impossible for them to commit them. Such persons do not fear there is some
superior being waiting to strike them to the earth
with a mighty club for doing certain things, simply
because that intelligence has laid down an apparently arbitrary law forbidding the commission of
the act. On the contrary they know that the higher
intelligences are possessed of nothing but intense

love for all living creatures, and are willing and ready to always help them, so far as is possible under the workings of the law. But such persons recognize the folly of the act, and therefore refrain from committing it—in fact, they have lost the desire to commit it. It is almost exactly parallel to the example of the child and the stove. A child who wants to touch the stove will do so as soon as he finds an opportunity, notwithstanding the commands of the parent, and in spite of threatened punishment. But let that child once experience the pain of the burn, and recognize that there is a close connection between a hot stove and a burnt finger, and it will keep away from the stove. The loving parent would like to protect its child from the result of its own follies, but the child-nature insists upon learning certain things by experience, and the parent is unable to prevent it. In fact, the child who is too closely watched and restrained, usually "breaks out" later in life, and learns certain things by itself. All that the parent is able to do is to surround the child with the ordinary safeguards, and to give it the benefit of his wisdom, a portion of which the child will store away—and then trust to the law of life to work out the result.

And so the human soul is constantly applying the test of experience to all phases of life—passing from one incarnation to another, constantly learning new lessons, and gaining new wisdom. Sooner or later it finds out how hurtful certain courses of action are—discovers the folly of certain actions and ways of living, and like the burnt child avoids those things in the future. All of us know that certain things "are no temptation to us," for we have learned the lesson at some time in some past life and do not need to re-learn it—while other things tempt us sorely, and we suffer much pain by reason thereof. Of what use would all this pain and sorrow be if this one life were all? But we carry the benefit of our experience into another life, and avoid the pain there. We may look around us and wonder why certain of our acquaintances cannot see the folly of certain forms of action, when it is so plain to us—but we forget that we have passed through just the same stage of experience that they are now undergoing, and have outlived the desire and ignorance—we do not realize that in future lives these people will be free from this folly and pain, for they will have learned the lesson by experience, just as have we.

It is hard for us to fully realize that we are what we are just by the result of our experiences. Let us take one single life as an example. You think that you would like to eliminate from your life some painful experience, some disgraceful episode; some mortifying circumstances; but have you ever stopped to think that if it were possible to eradicate these things, you would, of necessity, be forced to part with the experience and knowledge that has come to you from these occurrences. Would you be willing to part with the knowledge and experience that has come to you in the way mentioned? Would you be willing to go back to the state of inexperience and ignorance in which you were before the thing happened? Why, if you were to go back to the old state, you would be extremely likely to commit the same folly over again. How many of us would be willing to completely wipe out the experiences which have come to us? We are perfectly willing to forget the occurrence, but we know that we have the resulting experience built into our character, and we would not be willing to part with it, for it would be taking away a portion of our mental structure. If we were to part with experience gained through pain we would first part with one bit of ourselves, and then with another, until at last we would have nothing left except the mental shell of our former self.

But, you may say, of what use are the experiences gained in former lives, if we do not remember them—they are lost to us. But they are not lost to you—they are built into your mental structure, and nothing can ever take them away from you—they are yours forever. Your character is made up not only of your experiences in this particular life, but also of the result of your experiences in many other lives and stages of existence. You are what you are to-day by reason of these accumulated experiences—the experiences of the past lives and of the present one. You remember some of the things in the present life which have built up your character—but many others equally important, in the present life, you have forgotten—but the result stays with you, having been woven into your mental being. And though you may remember but little, or nothing, of your past lives, the experiences gained in them continue with you, now and forever. It is these past experiences which give you "predispositions" in certain directions — which make it very difficult for you to do certain things, and easy to do others—which cause you to "instinctively" recognize certain things as unwise or wrong, and to cause you to turn your back upon them as follies. They give you your "tastes" and inclinations, and make some ways seem better than others to you. Nothing is lost in life, and all the experiences of the past contribute to your well-being in the present—all your troubles and pains of the present will bear fruit in the future.

We do not always learn a lesson at one trial, and we are sent back to our task over and over again, until we have accomplished it. But not the slightest effort is ever lost, and if we have failed at the task in the past, it is easier for us to accomplish it to-day.

An American writer, Mr. Berry Benson, in the *Century Magazine,* of May, 1894, gives us a beautiful illustration of one of the features of the workings of the law of Spiritual Evolution. We reprint it, herewith:

"A little boy went to school. He was very little. All that he knew he had drawn in with his mother's milk. His teacher (who was God) placed him in the lowest class, and gave him these lessons to learn: Thou shalt not kill. Thou shalt do no hurt to any living thing. Thou shalt not steal. So the man did not kill; but he was cruel, and he stole. At the end of the day (when his beard was gray—when the night was come) his teacher (who was God) said: Thou hast learned not to kill, but the other lessons thou hast not learned. Come back tomorrow.

"On the morrow he came back a little boy. And his teacher (who was God) put him in a class a little higher, and gave him these lessons to learn: Thou shalt do no hurt to any living thing. Thou shalt not steal. Thou shalt not cheat. So the man did no hurt to any living thing; but he stole and he cheated. And at the end of the day (when his beard was gray—when the night was come) his teacher (who was God) said: Thou hast learned to be merciful. But the other lessons thou hast not learned. Come back tomorrow.

"Again, on the morrow, he came back, a little boy. And his teacher (who was God) put him in a class yet a little higher, and gave him these lessons to learn: Thou shalt not steal. Thou shalt not cheat. Thou shalt not covet. So the man did not steal; but he cheated and he coveted. And at the end of the day (when his beard was gray—when the night was come) his teacher (who was God) said: Thou hast learned not to steal. But the other lessons thou hast not learned. Come back, my child, tomorrow.

"This is what I have read in the faces of men

and women, in the book of the world, and i
scroll of the heavens, which is writ with star;

The great lesson to be learned by every so , ₃
the truth of the Oneness of All. This knowledge
carries with it all the rest. It causes one to follow
the precept of the Son of Mary, who said: "And
thou shalt love the Lord, thy God, with all thy
heart, and with all thy soul, and with all thy mind,
and with all thy strength;" and "Thou shalt love
thy neighbor as thyself." When man grows into a
consciousness of the truth that All is One—that
when one loves God he is loving the Whole Thing
—that his neighbor is indeed himself—then he has
but a few more classes to pass through before he
passes into the "High School" of Spiritual Knowledge. This conviction of the Oneness of All, carries with it certain rules of action—of divine ethics
—which transcend all written or spoken human
laws. The Fatherhood of God and the Brotherhood of Man become a reality rather than a mere
repetition of meaningless words. And this great
lesson must be learned by all—and all are learning
it by degrees. And this is the aim of the present
stage of Spiritual Evolution—to know God as He
is; to know your relationship with others—to know
what *we* are. There are greater schools, colleges
and universities of spiritual knowledge beyond us,
but these truths are the lessons taught in the grades
in which we are at present. And all this pain, and
trouble and sorrow, and work, has been but to
teach us these truths—but the truth once gained

is seen to be well worth even the great price paid for it.

If you ask the Yogis what is one's duty toward God (meaning God in the grandest conception of Him) they will answer "Love Him, and the rest will be made clear to you—and to know him is to Love him, therefore learn to Know Him." And if you ask them what is one's duty toward his fellow-men they will answer, simply: "*Be Kind*— and you will be all the rest." These two precepts, if followed, will enable one to live the Perfect Life. They are simple, but they contain all that is worth knowing concerning one's relations with the Infinite Power and with one's fellow-men. All the rest is froth and sediment—the worthless rubbish which has accumulated around the Divine Flame of the Truth. We mention them in this place, because they sum up the idea of the consciousness which all the race is striving hard to acquire. If you are able to make them a part of yourself, you will have made great progress on the Path—will have passed the Great Examination.

The doctrine of Spiritual Cause and Effect is based upon the great truth that under the Law each man is, practically, the master of his own destiny—his own judge—his own rewarder—his own awarder of punishment. That every thought, word or action, has its effect upon the future life or lives of the man—not in the nature of a reward or punishment (as these words are generally understood) as the inevitable result of the great Law of

cause and effect. The operation of the Law in surrounding us with certain sets of conditions in a new
birth, is influenced by two great general principles:
(1) The prevailing desires, aspirations, likes and
dislikes, and longing of the individual at that particular stage of his existence, and (2) By the influence of the unfolding Spirit, which, pressing
forward eagerly for fuller expression and less restraint, brings to bear upon the reincarnating soul
an influence which causes it to be governed in its
selection of the desirable conditions of its new
birth. Upon the apparently conflicting influences
of these two great forces rests the whole matter
of the circumstances and conditions surrounding
the rebirth of the soul, and also many of the conditions surrounding the personality in the new life
—for these conditions are governed greatly all
through life by these conflicting (or apparently
conflicting) forces.

The urge of the desires, aspirations, and habits
of the past life, is strongly pressing the soul towards incarnation in conditions best fitted for the
expression and manifestation of these likes, tastes
and desires—the soul wishes to go on along the line
of its past life, and naturally seeks circumstances
and surroundings best fitted for the freest expression
of its personality. But, at the same time, the Spirit,
within the soul, knows that the soul's unfoldment
needs certain other conditions to bring out certain
parts of its nature which have been suppressed or
not developed, and so it exerts an attraction upon

the reincarnating soul, drawing it a bit aside from its chosen course, and influencing that choice to a certain degree. A man may have an overpowering desire for material wealth, and the force of his desire will cause him to choose circumstances and conditions for a rebirth into a family where there is much wealth, or into a body best suited for the attainment of his desires, but the Spirit, knowing that the soul has neglected the development of kindness, will draw it a little aside, and cause it to be brought into the sweep of circumstances which will result in the man being made to suffer pain, disappointment and loss, even though he attain great wealth in his new life, to the end that he may develop that part of his nature.

We may see illustrations of this last mentioned occurrence in some of the very rich men of America. They have been born into circumstances in which they have had the freest expression of the desire for material wealth—they have possessed themselves of faculties best adapted to that one end, and have managed to be surrounded with circumstances best calculated to give the freest manifestations of those faculties. They have attained their heart's desire, and have piled up wealth in a manner unknown to former ages. But yet they are most unhappy and dissatisfied as a rule. Their wealth is a weight around their neck, and they are tormented by fears of losing it and the anxiety of attending to it. They feel that it has brought them no real happiness, but has on the contrary separated them from their fellow-men, and from the happiness known to those of moderate means. They are feverish and restless and constantly on the search for some new excitement which will divert their minds from the contemplation of their real condition. They feel a sense of their duty toward the race and although they do not quite understand the feeling behind it all, they endeavor to balance matters by contributing to colleges, hospitals, charities, and other similar institutions which have sprung up in response to the awakening consciousness of the race to the reality of the Brotherhood of Man and the Oneness of All. Before the end comes, they will feel in the depths of their soul that this success has not brought them real happiness, and in the period of rest which will follow their departure from the physical body, they will "take stock" of themselves, and readjust their mental and spiritual affairs, so that when they are again born they will no longer devote their entire energies toward the piling up of wealth that they cannot use, but will live a more balanced life, and will find happiness in unexpected quarters and will develop more spiritually. This is not because they have been impressed with the sense of any special "wickedness" in abnormal money getting, but because the soul has found that it did not secure happiness in that way, and is seeking elsewhere for it, and because it has lived out the desire for wealth, and has turned its attention to other things. Had the Spirit not exerted its influence, the man might have been born into the conditions tending to produce wealth, and yet not have been made to see the one-sidedness of such a life, in which case it would have continued to be possessed of such an abnormal desire for wealth that it would have been born again and again, with increasing power each time, until it would have become practically a money demon. But the Spirit's influence always counteracts abnormal desires, although sometimes several incarnations have to be lived through before the soul wears out its desire, and begins to be influenced by the Spirit to a marked extent. Sometimes the Spirit's influence is not sufficiently strong to prevent rebirth into conditions greatly favoring old desires, but in such cases it is often able to manage affairs during the life of the man, so as to teach him the lesson needed to call a halt upon his unbridled desires, by bringing him into the sweep of the Law of Attraction and causing certain pain to befall him—certain disappointment—certain failures—that will cause him to realize the pain, disappointment, failures and sorrow of others, and to bring upon him a course of living which will help to unfold his higher faculties. Many of the sudden strokes of "misfortune" are really brought about by this higher principle of the man, in order to teach him certain lessons for his own good. It is not necessarily a higher power which makes a man realize these lessons of life, but it is generally his own higher self — the Spirit within him — which brings about these results. The Spirit knows what is really best for the man, and when it sees his lower nature running away with him, tries to swing him from his course, or to bring him to a sudden stop if necessary. This is not as a punishment, remember, but as the greatest kindness. The Spirit is a part of that man, and not an outside power—although it is of course the Divine part of him—that part of him in nearest touch with the great over-ruling Intelligence which we call God. This pain is not brought about because of any feeling of righteous indignation, revenge, impatience or any similar feeling on the part of the Spirit, but is akin to the feeling of the most loving parent, who is forced to take from the hands of the little child some dangerous thing which may injure the little one—it is the hand which draws back the child from the brink of the precipice, although the little one screams with rage and disappointment because its desires are frustrated.

The man or woman in whom the Spiritual Mind is developed, sees this condition of things, and instead of fighting against the Spirit, yields himself or herself to it without friction, and obeys its guiding hand, and is thus saved much pain. But those who know not, rage and rebel at the restraining and guiding hand, strike at it, and attempt to tear away from it, thereby bringing upon themselves bitter experience made necessary by their rebellion. We are so apt to resent outside influence in our affairs that this idea of restraint is not pleasant to us, but if we will only remember that it is a part of *our-selves* — the higher part of us — that is doing this directing, then we may see the thing in a different light. And we must remember this: That no matter how adverse circumstances or conditions seem to be for us, they are exactly what we need under just the circumstances of our lives, and have for their only object our ultimate good. We may need strengthening along certain lines, in order to round us out—and we are apt to get just the experiences calculated to round out that particular part of us. We may be tending too much in one direction, and we are given a check and an urge in another direction. These little things—and great things all mean something. And then our interests are bound up more or less with those of others, owing to the laws of attraction, and our acts may be intended to reflect upon them, and theirs upon us, for our mutual development and ultimate good. We will have more to say on this subject a little later on.

If we will stand still, and calmly consider our past life (the present life, we mean) we will see that certain things have led to certain other things, and that small things have led to great things—that little turning points have resulted in an entire change in our life. We may trace back the most important thing in our life to some trifling incident or occurrence. We are able to look back and see how the painful experiences of the past have strengthened us, and have brought us to a larger and fuller life. We are able to see how that particular thing in the past, which seemed needlessly cruel and uncalled for, was the very thing which has brought us to some great thing in the present. All that is needed is the perspective of years. And if we get so that we are able to see this, we will be able to bear with a far greater degree of philosophy the pains and disagreeable occurrences of the present, knowing that they mean ultimate good. When we cease to think of these things as punishment, or a wanton interference of some outside power, or the cruelty of Nature, and begin to see them as either the consequences of our own past lives, or the result of the Spirit's directing hand, we will cease to protest and struggle as we have been doing in the past, and will endeavor to fall in with the working of the great Law, and will thereby avoid friction and pain. And no matter what pain, sorrow or trouble we may be undergoing, if we will open ourselves to the guidance of the Spirit, a way will be opened out for us—one step at a time—and if we follow it we will obtain peace and strength. The Law does not heap upon a back more than it can bear, and not only does it temper the wind to the shorn lamb, but tempers the shorn lamb to the wind.

We have spoken of our interests being bound up with those of others. This also is a principle of the law of Spiritual Cause and Effect. In our past lives we have attached ourselves to certain others, either by love or hate—either by kind action or by cruelty. And these people in this life have certain relation-

ships to us, all tending toward mutual adjustment
and mutual advancement and development. It is
not a law of revenge, but simply the law of cause
and effect which causes us to receive a hurt (when
a hurt is needed) from the hands of some one
whom we have hurt in some past life—and it is not
merely a law of reward for good, but that same law
of cause and effect, that causes some one to bind up
our wounds and comfort us, whom we have com-
forted and helped in some past life. The person
who is caused to hurt us, may have no intention of
doing so, being a perfectly innocent party, but we
are brought into conditions whereby we receive
pain from the acts of that person, although he be
unconscious of it. If he hurts us consciously, and
still in obedience to the law, it is because he is still
on that plane, and is willing to hurt us, and is
brought by the Law of Attraction into a condition
whereby we may receive hurt from him. But even
that hurt is calculated to benefit us, in the end, so
wonderful is this law of cause and effect consti-
tuted. Of course, if we once reach the position
where we see the truth, we do not need so many of
these lessons, and their necessity having passed, the
law allows us to escape that which would otherwise
have given us pain.

The above mentioned condition of affairs may
be illustrated by the case of one who in a past
incarnation deliberately won the love of another,
for selfish reasons, and then having gratified the
desire willfully threw aside the other one, as one

would a worn-out toy. While not pretending to explain the exact working of the law in any particular case, we have been informed by those who have watched these matters from a higher point of view, that in such a case as above mentioned, the betrayer would probably in this life, fall violently in love with the person who was the victim in the last life, but the latter would be utterly unable to return that affection, and the former would suffer all the pain that comes to one who loves in vain, the result being that he would be brought to a realization of the sacredness of human affection, and the unkindness of trifling with it. It will be noticed in this case that the person causing pain in the present life is a perfectly innocent party to the whole thing and thereby does not start new causes and effects.

Those whom we have loved and have been friendly to in past lives are very apt to be connected with our present life, being kept near us by the law of attraction. The people who are brought into close relations with us are, in all probability, those with whom we have been close in past lives. Sudden likes and dislikes, so often observed between people, may be accounted for on this theory of rebirth, and many of the occurrences of our every day lives come under this law of spiritual cause and effect. We are constantly bound up with the lives of others, for pain or happiness, and the law must work out its course. The only escape from the complete working out of the law is the acquirement of the knowledge of the truth on our part, and the consequent modeling of our lives on the lines of this higher truth, in which case we are relieved of the unnecessary lessons, and we ride on the top of the wave, instead of having it submerge us.

Let us beware how we start into operation this law of cause and effect by Hate, Malice, Jealousy, Anger, and general Unkindness toward others. Let us be as Kind as we can, in all justice to ourselves and others, and let us avoid feelings of Hate and a desire for Revenge. Let us live on, bearing our burdens with as much grace as we can summon, and let us always trust in the guidance of the Spirit, and the help of the highest Intelligence. Let us know that all is working together for good, and that we cannot be deprived of that good. Let us remember that this life is as but a grain of sand in the desert of time, and that we have long ages ahead of us, in which we will have a chance to work out all our aspirations and high desires. Be not discouraged for God reigns, and all is well.

THE FOURTEENTH LESSON.

THE YOGI PATH OF ATTAINMENT.

The student who has carefully acquainted himself with the fundamental principles of the Yogi Philosophy, as set forth in these lessons, will readily see that anyone who grasps and accepts these teachings, and makes them a part of his everyday life, will naturally live a very different life from one to whom this present earth-life is all, and who believes that death extinguishes individuality, and that there is no future life or lives. It will also lead one to live his life rather differently from the person who believes that we are but creatures of a rather capricious Providence, having but little responsibility of our own, and that our "salvation" depends upon a perfunctory "belief" in certain teachings, and a set form of attendance at certain forms of religious worship. Remember, now, please, that the Yogi Philosophy has no fault to find with *any* form of religion—it teaches that *all* forms of religion are good, and each has its particular place to fill—each fills the need of humanity in some of its stages. It believes that no matter what form of worship is followed—no matter what conception of Deity is held—that every man really worships the

One Great Intelligence, which we know under many names, and that the varying forms of such worship are immaterial, the motive behind each being the real test to be applied.

But the Yogi Philosophy, and, in fact, the teachings of all occultists, to whatever race they may belong, or what particular creed may be favored by them, hold that man is a responsible being, that he really makes his own conditions and bestows his own rewards and punishments, as a natural consequence of his acts. It also teaches that man cannot escape his own good, and that though he may slip backward a hundred times, still will he always make some little progress, and in the end will conquer his material nature, and then move steadily forward to the great goal. It teaches that we are all God's children, no matter what form of worship we may favor—that there are none of God's children destined to be utterly cut off or damned. It teaches that we are punished *by* our sins instead of *for* them, and that the law of cause and effect brings its inevitable result. It emphasizes the teachings that "as we sow so shall we reap," and shows just how and why we reap what we have sown. It shows how our lower desires and passions will weigh us down, and surround us with environments that will cause us to outlive them, and make us so thoroughly sick and tired of them that the soul will, eventually, recoil in horror from its past life of material grossness, and in so doing will receive an impetus in the right direction. It shows us that we have the Spirit always with us, anxious and willing to give us help and guidance, and that, through the Spirit, we are always in close connection with the source of all life and power.

Men are of varying temperaments, and the course that will best suit one will not be adapted to the requirements of another. One will seek progress and development in one direction, and another in a different way, and a third by a still different course. The Yogi Philosophy teaches that the way that seems to appeal the most to a man's general temperament and disposition is the one best adapted to his use at the present time. They divide the Path of Attainment into three paths leading up to the great main road. They call these three paths, (1) Raja Yoga; (2) Karma Yoga; (3) Gnani Yoga; each of these forms of Yoga being a path leading to the Great Road, and each being traveled by those who may prefer it—but all lead to the same place. In this lesson we will give a brief description of each of the three paths, which together are known to the Yogis as "The Threefold Path."

Some of the teachers treat what is known as "Bhakti Yoga" as if it were a separate path, but we prefer thinking of it as being an incident of each of the three paths, as "Bhakti Yoga" is really what we might call the "religious" form of Yoga, teaching the love and worship of God, according to how he appears to us through the colored glasses of our own particular creed. We fail to see how one may follow any of the several Yoga paths without being filled with love and reverence for the great Centre of all Life—the Absolute—God—by whatever name we know it. The term "Bhakti Yoga" really means the "way of devotion." Let us trust that all our students, no matter which of the three paths they may elect to follow, will carry with them the devotion inculcated in the "Bhakti Yoga" of the particular religious body with which they are affiliated, and not feel that the "Threefold Path" calls for their renouncing that which has been dear to them from childhood. On the contrary, we think that a careful study of the Yogi Philosophy will awaken a new interest in religion, and cause many to understand much that they formerly but blindly "believed," and will cause them to develop a deeper religious spirit, rather than a lesser one.

"Raja Yoga" is devoted to the development of the latent powers in Man—the gaining of the control of the mental faculties by the Will—the attainment of the mastery of the lower self—the development of the mind to the end that the soul may be aided in its unfoldment. It teaches as its first step the care and control of the body, as taught in "Hatha Yoga," holding that the body should be rendered an efficient instrument, and under good control, before the best results may be attained along mental and psychic lines. Much that the Western World has been attracted to in late years under the name of "Mental Science" and similar terms, really comes under the head of "Raja Yoga." This form of Yoga recognizes the wonderful power of the trained mind and will, and the marvelous results that may be gained by the training of the same, and its application by concentration, and intelligent direction. It teaches that not only may the mind be directed outward, influencing outside objects and things, but that it may also be turned inward, and concentrated upon the particular subject before us, to the end that much hidden knowledge may be unfolded and uncovered. Many of the great inventors are really practicing "Raja Yoga" unconsciously, in this inward application of it, while many leaders in the world of affairs are making use of its outward, concentrated application in their management of affairs.

But the follower of the "Raja Yoga" path is not content alone with the attainment of powers for either of the above uses. He seeks still greater heights, and manages by the same, or similar processes, to turn the searchlight of concentrated mind into his own nature, thus bringing to light many hidden secrets of the soul. Much of the Yogi Philosophy has really been brought to light in this way. The practice of "Raja Yoga" is eminently practical, and is in the nature of the study and practice of chemistry—it proves itself as the student takes each step. It does not deal in vague theories, but teaches experiments and facts from first to last. We hope to be able to give to our students, in the near future, a practical work on the subject of "Hatha Yoga," for which work there seems to be a great need in the Western world, which seems to be waiting to be told "how" to do those things which have been stated to be possible by numerous writers who had grasped the theory but had not acquainted themselves with the practice accompanying the theory.

"Karma Yoga" is the "Yoga" of Work. It is the path followed by those who delight in their work—who take a keen interest in "doing things" with head or hand — those who believe in work "for work's sake." "Karma" is the Sanscrit word applied to the "Law of Spiritual Cause and Effect," of which we have spoken in a preceding lesson. "Karma Yoga" teaches how one may go through life working—and taking an interest in action—without being influenced by selfish consideration, which might create a fresh chain of cause and effect which would bind him to objects and things, and thus retard his spiritual progress. It teaches "work for work's sake" rather than from a desire for results. Strange as this may seem to many of our Western readers, it is a fact that many of the men of the Western world who have accomplished much, have really been possessed of this idea, without realizing it and have really worked for the joy of the action and creative effort, and have really cared but little for the fruit of their labors. Some of them say that they "have worked because they could not help it," rather than from the mere desire for material gain. The follower of "Karma Yoga," seems to himself, at times, as if he were not the real worker, but that his mind and body were doing the work, and he,—himself—were standing off and watching himself work or act. There are lower and higher phases of "Karma Yoga", which cannot be explained here, as each branch of Yoga is a great subject in itself.

"Gnani Yoga" is the "Yoga" of Wisdom. It is followed by those of a scientific, intellectual type, who are desirous of reasoning out, proving, experimenting, and classifying the occult knowledge. It is the path of the scholar. Its follower is strongly attracted toward metaphysics. Examples of the idea of "Gnani Yogi"—apparently widely differing examples—are to be seen in the great philosophers of ancient and modern times, and in the other extreme, those who have a strong tendency toward metaphysical teachings. As a matter of fact, nearly all students of the Yogi Philosophy are more or less attracted to "Gnani Yoga", even though they be said to be following one of the other of the three paths. These lessons, for instance, are a part of the "Gnani Yoga" work, although they are combined with other forms of Yoga. Many Yogis combine in themselves the attributes of the followers of several forms of Yoga, although their natural tendencies cause them to favor one of the paths more than the others.

Of the three forms of Yoga, the second, or "Karma Yoga" is perhaps the easiest one to follow, for the student. It requires less study, and less practice—less of the research of "Gnani Yoga", and less of the training of "Raja Yoga." The Karma Yogi simply tries to lead a good life, doing his work to the best of his ability, without being carried away with the hope of reward—he grows into a realization of the truth regarding his nature, and is content to gradually unfold, like a rose, from life to life, until he reaches a high stage of attainment. He does not long for unusual powers, and consequently does not endeavor to develop them. He does not long for the solution of the great problems of nature and life, but is content to live on, one day at a time, knowing and trusting that all will be well with him—and it will. Many of the "New Thought" people of America, are really Karma Yogis. The Raja Yogi, on the contrary, feels a desire to develop his latent powers and to make researches into his own mind. He wishes to manifest hidden powers and faculties, and feels a keen longing to experiment along these lines. He is intensely interested in psychology and "psychic phenomena", and all occult phenomena and teachings along similar lines. He is able to accomplish much by determined effort, and often manifests wonderful results by means of the concentrated will and mind. The Gnani Yogi's chief pleasure consists in metaphysical reasoning, or subtle intellectual research. He is the philosopher; scholar; preacher; teacher; student; and often goes to extreme lengths in following his favorite line of work, losing sight of the other sides of the subject.

The man best calculated to make general advancement along occult lines is the one who avoids running to extremes in any one of the branches of the subject, but who, while in the main following his own inclinations toward certain forms of "Yoga", still keeps up a general acquaintance with the several phases of the great philosophy. In the end, man must develop on all his many sides, and why not keep in touch with all sides while we journey along. By following this course we avoid one-sidedness; fanaticism; narrowness; short-sightedness, and bigotry.

Yogi students may be divided into three general classes: (1) Those who have made considerable progress along the same lines, in past incarnations, and who have awakened to consciousness in the present life with the strongest tendencies toward occultism and similar subjects. These people learn rapidly and are conscious of the fact that they are but relearning some lesson learned in the past. They grasp occult truths intuitively and find in such studies food for the hunger of the soul. These souls are, of course, in various stages of development. Some have but an elementary acquaintance with the subject, their knowledge in the past incarnation having been but slight; others have progressed further, and are able to go much further in their present work than those who are less developed; still others are quite highly developed, and lack but little of having reached the "conscious" stage of incarnation, that is, the state of being able to awaken to a conscious knowledge of past lives. The last mentioned sub-class are apt to be regarded as "queer" by their associates, particularly in early life—they appear "old" and "strange" to their companions. They feel as if they were strangers in a strange land, but sooner or later are sure to be brought into contact with others, or made acquainted with teachings, which will enable them to take up their studies again.

(2) Those who awaken to a conscious knowledge, to a greater or lesser degree, of their past lives, and what they have learned there. Such people are comparatively rare, and yet there are far more of them than is generally supposed, for these people are not apt to bestow their confidence upon chance acquaintances, and generally regard their knowledge and memory of the past as something sacred. These people go through the world, sowing a little seed here, and a little there, which seed falling on fertile ground bears fruit in the future incarnations of those who receive them.

(3) Those who have heard some occult truths in past incarnations—some words of wisdom, knowledge or advice dropped by some of those who have advanced further along the path. In their mental soil, if rich, they let these seed-thoughts sink deep into them, and in the next life the plant appears. These people are possessed of an unrest, which makes them dissatisfied with the current explanations of things, and which causes them to search here and there for the truth, which they intuitively know is to be found somewhere. They are often led to run after false prophets, and from one teacher to another, gaining a little truth here, having an error

corrected there. Sooner or later they find an anchorage, and in their rest they lay up stores of knowledge, which (after being digested in the period of soul-rest in the Astral World) will be of great value to them in their next incarnation.

It will be readily recognized that it is practically impossible to give detailed directions suited for the varying needs of these different students. All that can be done (outside of personal instruction from some competent teacher) is to give words of general advice and encouragement. But do not let this discourage you. Remember this—*it is a great occult truth*—when the student is ready the teacher appears—the way will be opened to you step by step, and as each new spiritual need comes into existence, the means to satisfy it will be on the way. It may come from without—it may come from within—but come it *will.* Do not let discouragement creep over you because you seem to be surrounded by the most unfavorable environments, with no one near to whom you can talk of these great truths that are unfolding before your mental vision. This isolation is probably just what you need in order to make you self-reliant and to cure you of that desire to lean upon some other soul. We have these lessons to learn—and many others—and the way that seems hardest for us to travel is very often the one laid out for us, in order that we may learn the needed lesson well and "for good."

It follows that one who has grasped the fundamental ideas of this philosophy will begin to find

Fear dropping from him—for when he realizes just what he is, how can he fear? There being nothing that is able to really hurt him, why should he fear? Worry, of course, follows after Fear, and when Fear goes, many other minor mental faults follow after it. Envy, Jealousy and Hate — Malice, Uncharitableness and Condemnation—cannot exist in the mind of one who "understands". Faith and Trust in the Spirit, and that from which the Spirit comes, must be manifest to the awakened soul. Such a one naturally recognizes the Spirit's guidance, and unhesitatingly follows it, with fear—without doubt. Such a one cannot help being Kind—to him the outside world of people seem to be as little children (many of them like babes unborn) and he deals with them charitably, not condemning them in his heart, for he knows them for what they are. Such a one performs the work which is set before him, knowing that such work, be it humble or exalted, has been brought to him by his own acts and desires, or his needs—and that it is all right in any event, and is but the stepping-stone to greater things. Such a one does not fear Life—does not fear Death—both seem as but differing manifestations of the same thing—one as good as the other.

The student who expects to make progress, must make his philosophy a part of his every day life. He must carry it around with him always. This does not mean that he should thrust his views and opinions upon others—in fact, that is expressly contrary to occult teachings, for no one has the right to force opinions upon others, and it is contrary to natural growth and freedom of the individual soul. But the student should be able to carry with him an abiding sense of the reality and truth of his philosophy. He need not be afraid to take it with him *anywhere,* for it fits into all phases of life. If one cannot take it with him to work, something is wrong with either the philosophy or the work, or the individual. And it will help us to work better —to do more earnest work—for we know that the work is necessary for the development of some part of us—otherwise it would not be set before us— and no matter how disagreeable the task, we may be able to sing with joy when we realize just what we are and what great things are before us. The slave chained to the galley—if he have peace in his soul and the knowledge in his mind—is far less to be pitied than the king on his throne who lacks these things. We must not shirk our tasks, not run away from our destiny—for we cannot really get rid of them except by performing them. And these very disagreeable things are really strengthening our character, if we are learning our lesson aright. And then, remember "even these things shall pass away."

One of the greatest hindrances to the progress of the student into the higher stages of occultism, particularly the phenomenal phases, is the lack of self-control. When one wishes to be placed in possession of power, which, if carelessly used or misused, may result in the hurt of oneself or others, it is the greatest importance that such a one should have attained the mastery of self—the control of the emotional side of his nature. Imagine a man possessed of high occult powers losing his temper and flying into a rage, sending forth vibrations of Hate and Anger intensified by the increased force of his developed powers. Such exhibitions, in a man who has attained occult powers, would be very harmful to him, as they would, perhaps, be manifested upon a plane where such things have an exaggerated effect. A man whose investigations lead him on to the Astral Plane, should beware of such a loss of self-control, as a failing of this kind might be fatal to him. But, so nicely is the world of the higher forces balanced that a man of violent temper, or one who lacks self-control, can make but little progress in occult practices — this being a needed check. So one of the first things to be accomplished by the student who wishes to advance is the mastery of his emotional nature and the acquirement of self-control.

A certain amount of courage of the higher sort is also needed, for one experiences some strange sights and happenings on the astral plane, and those who wish to travel there must have learned to master fear. One also needs calmness and poise. When we remember that worry and kindred emotions cause vibrations around us, it may readily be seen that such conditions of mind are not conducive to psychical research—in fact the best results cannot be obtained when these things are present.

The occultist who wishes to attain great powers must first purge himself of selfish grasping for these things for the gratification of his own base ends, for the pursuit of occult powers with this desire will bring only pain and disappointment and the one who attempts to prostitute psychic power for base ends will bring upon himself a whirlwind of undesirable results. Such forces, when misused, react as a boomerang upon the sender. The true occultist is filled with love and brotherly feeling for his fellow men, and endeavors to aid them instead of to beat them down in their progress.

Of all the numerous books written for the purpose of throwing light on the path of the student of occultism, we know of none better fitted for the purpose than that wonderful little book called "Light on the Path", written down by "M. C.", at the instigation of some intelligences far above the ordinary. It is veiled in the poetic style common to the Orientals, and at first glance may seem paradoxical. But it is full of the choicest bits of occult wisdom, for those who are able to read it. It must be read "between the lines", and it has a peculiarity that will become apparent to any one who may read it carefully. That is, it will give you as much truth as you are able to grasp to-day; and tomorrow when you pick it up it will give you more, from the same lines. Look at it a year from now, and new truths will burst upon you—and so on, and on. It contains statements of truth so wonderfully stated —and yet half-concealed—that as you advance in spiritual discernment—and are ready for greater truths each day—you will find that in this book veil after veil will be lifted from before the truth, until you are fairly dazzled. It is also remarkable as a book which will give consolation to those in trouble or sorrow. Its words (even though they be but half-understood) will ring in the ears of its readers, and like a beautiful melody will soothe and comfort and rest those who hear it. We advise all of our students to read this little book often and with care. They will find that it will describe various spiritual experiences through which they will pass, and will prepare them for the next stage. Many of our students have asked us to write a little book in the way of an elementary explanation of "Light on the Path"—perhaps the Spirit may lead us to do so at some time in the future—perhaps not.

It is not without a feeling of something like sadness that we write these concluding lines. When we wrote our First Lesson, we bade our students be seated for a course of talks—plain and simple— upon a great subject. Our aim was to present these great truths in a plain, practical simple manner, so that many would take an interest in them, and be led toward higher presentations of the truth. We have felt that love and encouragement, which is so necessary for a teacher, and have been assured of the sympathy of the Class from the first. But, on looking over our work it seems that we have said so little—have left unsaid so much—and yet we have done the best we could, considering the small space at our disposal and the immense field to be covered. We feel that we have really only begun, and yet it is now time to say "good-bye". Perhaps we have made some points a little clear to a few who have been perplexed—perhaps we have opened a door to those who were seeking entrance to the temple—who knows? If we have done even a little for only one person, our time has been well spent.

At some future time we may feel called upon to pass on to you a higher and more advanced presentation of this great subject—that is a matter which depends much upon your own desires—if you need us you will find us ready and willing to join you in the study of the great truths of the Yogi Philosophy. But, before you take the next step onward, be sure that you understand these elementary lessons thoroughly. Go over and over them, until your mind has fully grasped the principles. You will find new features presenting themselves with each reading. As your minds unfold, you will find new truths awaiting you even in the same pages that you have read and re-read several times. This, not because of any special merit in our work (for this work is crude, very crude, to our idea), but because of the inherent truth of the philosophy itself, which renders any thing written upon it to be filled with subject for thought and earnest consideration.

Good-bye dear students. We thank you for your kindness in listening to us during the term of this Class. We have felt your sympathy and love, as many of you must have felt ours. We feel sure that as you read these lines—filled with our earnest thoughts of kinship to you—you will feel our nearness to you in the Spirit—will be conscious of that warm hand-clasp which we extend to you across the miles that separate us in the flesh.

Remember these words, from *"Light on the Path"*: "When the disciple is ready to learn, then he is accepted, acknowledged, recognized. It must be so, for he has lit his lamp and it cannot be hidden."

Therefore, we say "Peace be with You."

FIRST LESSON—MANTRAM.

A mantram is a word, phrase, or verse used by the Eastern people in order to concentrate upon an idea and to let it sink deep into the mind. It is similiar to the "statements," or "affirmations," used by the Mental Scientists and others of the Western world.

The mantram for the month is a verse from a Western poet, Mr. Orr:

> "Lord of a thousand worlds am I,
> And I reign since time began;
> And night and day, in cyclic sway,
> Shall pass while their deeds I scan.
> Yet time shall cease, ere I find release,
> For I am the Soul of Man."

Commit this verse to memory, and repeat it often, letting the mind dwell upon the idea of immortality expressed so strongly, remembering always that YOU are the "I" referred to.

SECOND LESSON—MANTRAM.

"I AM MASTER OF MYSELF." Commit these words to memory, and repeat them often, letting the mind dwell upon the thoughts given in our Meditation for this month. Remember always that the "I" is the highest part of you that has been awakened into consciousness, and should, to a great extent be master of the animal nature from which you have emerged.

THIRD LESSON—MANTRAM.

The mantram for the month is the first verse of Cardinal Newman's hymn, "Lead, Kindly Light," which contains the deepest spiritual truth, but which is only imperfectly understood by the majority of the thousands who sing it. We trust that what we have said of Spirit will help you better to comprehend the hidden beauties of this grand old hymn:

"Lead, kindly Light, amid the encircling gloom
   Lead thou me on.
The night is dark, and I am far from home;
   Lead thou me on.
Keep thou my feet; I do not ask to see
The distant scene; one step enough for me.
   Lead thou me on."

FOURTH LESSON—MANTRAM.

The mantram for the month is: "I RADIATE THOUGHT WAVES OF THE KIND I DESIRE TO RECEIVE FROM OTHERS." This mantram conveys a mighty occult truth, and, if conscientiously repeated and lived up to, will enable you to make rapid progress in development and attainment. Give and you will receive—measure for measure—kind for kind—color for color. Your thought waves extend far beyond the visible aura, and affect others, and draw to you the thoughts of others corresponding in character and quality with those sent out by you. Thought is a living force—use it wisely.

FIFTH LESSON—MANTRAM AND MEDITATION.

The mantram for the month is: "Thought is a Living Force—I will use it wisely and well!"

Our subject for Meditation this month is our responsibility in the matter of adding to the world's thought. When we think that we are constantly adding to the supply of the world's thought, and also realize the enormous quantity of undeveloped thought which is being poured out from the minds of persons of a low order of development, we are led to a realization of our duty in the matter of helping to elevate and purify the volume of thought. We should guard ourselves against indulging in unworthy thoughts, and should try to radiate thoughts of help, comfort, cheer, and uplifting to our fellow-beings. Each of us can do his share of this work, and the help of each is needed. Send out thought-forms of help and love to your brothers and sisters—both in general and in particular. If you know of a struggling soul, send to it thoughts of comfort and encouragement. If you know of any in distress, send them thoughts of strength and help. Send forth your best helpful thought to the world. It may reach some fellow-being at a critical moment. When in distress yourself, there is no better way of receiving the help of strong thought of-others than to send forth hopeful thoughts to others who may be likewise distressed. We can help each other in this way, and will thus open up channels of communication which will be helpful to all. Misuse not the power of thought. Let this be your rule and standard: *Send no thought to another that you would not care to attract to yourself.* Peace be with you.

SIXTH LESSON—MANTRAM AND MEDITATION.

"Before the eyes can see, they must be incapable of tears. Before the ear can hear, it must have lost its sensitiveness. Before the voice can speak in the presence of the Masters, it must have lost the power to wound."

These words are capable of a number of meanings, each adapted to the wants of different people in various stages of development. They have their psychic meaning, their intellectual meaning, and their spiritual meaning. We take for our Meditation this month one of the many meanings. Let us take it into the Silence with us. Our eyes must be incapable of the tears of wounded pride; unkind criticisms; unmerited abuse; unfriendly remarks; the little annoyances of everyday life; the failures and disappointments of everyday existence before we can see clearly the great spiritual truths. Let us endeavor to rise, by degrees, above these incidents of personality, and strive to realize our individuality — the I Am — which is above the annoyances of personality, and to learn that these things cannot hurt the Real Self, and that they will be washed from the sands of time by the ocean of eternity. Likewise our ear must lose its sensitiveness to the unpleasant incidents of the personality (above alluded to as causing tears) before it can hear the truth clearly and free from the jarring noises of the outward strife of personality. One must grow to be able to hear these things and yet smile, secure in the knowledge of his soul and his powers, and destiny. Before the voice can speak to those high in the order of life and spiritual intelligence, it must have long since forgotten how to wound others by unkind words, petty spite, unworthy speech. The advanced man does not hesitate to speak the truth even when it is not pleasant, if it seems right to do so, but he speaks in the tone of a loving brother, who does not criticise, but merely feels the other's pain and wishes to remove its cause. Such a one has risen above the desire to "talk back" —to "cut" another by unkind and spiteful remarks, or to "get even" by saying, in effect: "You're another." These things must be cast aside like a worn-out cloak—the advanced man needs them not. Take these thoughts with you into the Silence, and let the truth sink into your mind, that it may take root, grow, blossom and bear fruit.

SEVENTH LESSON—MANTRAM AND MEDITATION.

"I Absorb from the Universal Supply of Energy, a sufficient Supply of Prana to Invigorate my Body—to Endow it with Health, Strength, Activity, Energy and Vitality."

The above Mantram and the following subjects for Meditation are designed to build up the physical body, in order to render it a more perfect instrument for the expression of life. Our previous Mantrams and Meditations have been designed for mental and spiritual development, but we realize that many are burdened by bodies manifesting inharmony and lack of perfect health, and we think it advisable to follow up this month's lesson Prana and Human Magnetism, with a Mantram and Meditation along the lines just mentioned.

Let the student place himself in a comfortable position, and after composing his mind, let him repeat the Mantram over a number of times until he experiences that peculiar rhythm and thrill that comes from such practice. Then let him concentrate upon the idea of the great supply of Pranic Energy in the Universe. The entire Universe is filled with this great Force—this great Life Principle—whereby all forms of motion, force and energy are made possible. Let him realize that he is free to draw upon it at will—that it is HIS OWN to use for the building up of the body—the Temple of the Spirit—and let him fear not to demand his own. Let him call for what is his, feeling certain that his just call will be answered. Let him breathe slowly, according to the instructions regarding the Rhythmic Breath (Science of Breath, pages 53-54) and mentally picture the inflow of Prana with each inward breath, and the expelling of worn out and impure matter with each outward breath. Let him picture himself as being filled with health, strength and vitality—full of energy and life—bright and happy.

If tired or fatigued during the day, let him stop for a moment and inhale a few deep breaths, carrying the mental picture of the inflowing Prana, and the casting out of diseased matter through the breath. He will find that he experiences an immediate feeling of increased strength and vitality. This Prana may be sent to any part of the body which seems to call for help and strength, and a little practice will enable the student to have such control that he can plainly feel the tingling sensation accompanying the passage of the Prana to the afflicted or tired part of the body. If one is lying down, the passing of the hands over one's body from the head downward with an occasional resting of the hands over the Solar Plexus, will be found beneficial and soothing. The hands may be easily charged with Prana by extending them loosely at full length and gently swinging them to and fro, and occasionally making a motion as if one was sprinkling water on something by throwing it off from the finger tips. A tingling sensation will be felt in the fingers and the whole hand will be so charged with Prana that it will relieve pain in other parts of the body, and in the bodies of others, if you desire to help them. Carry the thought of Health, Strength, Activity, Energy and Vitality into the Silence with you.

EIGHTH LESSON—MANTRAM AND MEDITATION.

"I am passing through this stage of existence making the best use of Head, Heart and Hand."

Each one of us here has his own work to do. We are here for a purpose, and until we fall in with the law and work out the tasks set before us, we will have these tasks constantly and repeatedly put before us until they are accomplished. The purpose of the accomplishment of these tasks is experience and growth, and, unpleasant as our tasks may seem, they have a most direct bearing upon our future growth and life. When we fall in with the workings of the law, and see and feel what is behind it, we cease to rebel and beat our heads against the wall. In opening up ourselves to the workings of the Spirit and being willing to work out our own salvation and accomplish our world's tasks, we really take the first step toward emancipation from the unpleasant tasks. When we cease to allow our work to be unpleasant to us, we find ourselves working into better things, as the lesson has been learned. Each person has placed before him just the work in the world best suited to his growth at that particular time—his wants have been consulted, and just the right thing allotted to him. There is no chance about this—it is the inexorable workings of the great law. And the only true philosophy consists in making up one's mind to do the work set before him to the best of his ability. As long as he shirks it, he will be kept to the task—when he begins to take a pleasure in doing it right, other things open up before him. To hate and fear a thing is to tie that thing to you. When you see it in its right relation—after your spiritual eyes are opened—then you begin to be freed from it.

And in going through Life—in doing our work in the world— we must make the best possible use of the three great gifts of the Spirit—the Head; the Heart; and the Hand. The Head (representing the intellectual part of our nature) must be given the opportunity to grow—it must be furnished the food upon which it thrives—it must not be cramped and starved—it must be used, as exercise strengthens and develops it. We must develop our minds, and not be afraid of thinking thoughts. The Mind must be kept free. The Heart (representing the love nature in its best sense) must be employed and must not be starved, chained or chided. We are not speaking of the lower forms of animal passion, miscalled Love, but of that higher thing belonging to the human race, which is a promise of greater things to come in the evolution of the race. It is that which begets sympathy, compassion, tenderness and kindness. It must not be allowed to sink to maudlin sentiment, but must be used in connection with the Head. It must reach out to embrace all Life in its enfolding embrace, and to feel that sense of kinship with all living things, which marks the man or woman of spiritual development. The Hand (representing the manifestation of physical creation and work) must be trained to do the work set before it the best it knows how. It must learn to do things well, and to feel that all work is noble and not degrading. It is the symbol of physical creation, and must be respected and honored. The man or woman of spiritual development goes through the world making the best use of Head, Heart and Hand.

NINTH LESSON—MANTRAM AND MEDITATION.

The Mantram for the month is " I AM."

When you say " I AM" you assert the reality of your existence— not the mere reality of the physical existence, which is but temporary and relative—but your real existence in the Spirit, which is not temporary or relative, but is eternal and absolute. You are asserting the reality of the Ego— the "I." The real "I" is not the body, but is the Spirit principle which is manifesting in body and mind. The real "I" is independent of the body, which is but a vehicle for its expression—it is indestructible and eternal. It cannot die nor become annihilated. It may change the form of its expression, or the vehicle of manifestation—but it is always the same "I"—a bit of the great ocean of Spirit—a spiritual atom manifesting in your present consciousness along the lines of spiritual unfoldment. Do not think of your soul as a thing apart from you, for YOU are the soul, and all the rest is transitory and changeable. Picture yourself in your mind as an entity apart from, and independent of, the body, which is but your shell—realize that it is possible for you to leave the body, and still be YOU. During a part of your period of meditation mentally ignore the body entirely, and you will find that you will gradually awaken to a sense of the independent existence of your soul—YOURSELF —and come to a consciousness of your real nature.

The student should endeavor to give a few moments each day to silent meditation, finding as quiet a place as possible, and then lying or sitting in an easy position, relaxing every muscle of the body and calming the mind. Then when the proper conditions are observed he will experience that peculiar sensation of calmness and quiet which will indicate that he is "entering the silence." Then he should dwell upon the subject given for meditation, repeating the Mantram in order to impress the meaning upon his mind. At such times he will receive more or less inspiration from his Spiritual Mind, and will feel stronger and freer all day.

The Mantram for this month, if clearly understood and impressed upon the consciousness, will give to the student an air of quiet dignity and calm manifestation of power which will have its effect upon people with whom he comes in contact. It will surround him with a thought aura of strength and power. It will enable him to cast off fear and to look the world of men and women calmly in the eyes, knowing that he is an eternal soul, and that naught can really harm him. A full realization of "I AM" will cause fear to fade away, for why should the Spirit fear anything?—nothing can harm it. We urge the cultivation of this state of consciousness upon our students. It will lift you above the petty worries, hates, fears, and jealousies of the lower mental states, and will cause you to be men and women "of the Spirit" in reality. You will find that the result will be felt by those with whom you come in contact. There is an undefinable aura surrounding these people of the "I AM" consciousness which causes them to be respected by the world around them.

The Complete Work

of

YOGI RAMACHARAKA

SCIENCE OF BREATH

FOURTEEN LESSONS YOGI PHILOSOPHY

ADVANCED COURSE IN YOGI PHILOSOPHY

RAJA YOGA

GNANI YOGA

PHILOSOPHIES AND RELIGIONS OF INDIA

HATHA YOGA

PSYCHIC HEALING

MYSTIC CHRISTIANITY

LIFE BEYOND DEATH

BHAGAVAD GITA

THE SPIRIT OF THE UPANISHADS

PRACTICAL WATER CURE

The Complete Works

of

YOGI RAMACHARAKA

—